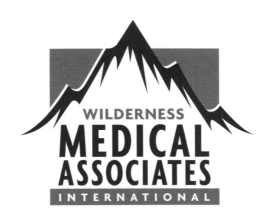

WILDERNESS AND RESCUE MEDICINE
WORKBOOK

Practical Case Studies for the Basic and Advanced Practitioner

Tom Clausing, WEMT-Paramedic

Contents

Abbreviations

ABC	Airway, Breathing, Circulation		PAS	Patient Assessment System
ABD	Abdomen		PCN	Penicillin
ALS	Advanced Life Support		PFA	Pain Free Activity
AMS	Acute Mountain Sickness		PI	Povidone Iodine
ASA	Aspirin		PO	By mouth
ASR	Acute Stress Reaction		prn	As needed
AVPU	Awake		Pt	Patient
	Verbal stimulus response		PPV	Positive Pressure Ventilation
	Painful stimulus response		PROP	Position
	Unresponsive			Reassurance
BLS	Basic Life Support			O2
$\overline{c}$	With			PPV
°C	Celcius		$\overline{q}$	Every
c/c	Chief Complaint		RICE	Rest
CHF	Congestive Heart Failure			Ice
cm	Centimeter			Compression
CNS	Central Nervous System			Elevation
c/o	Complains Of...		ROM	Range Of Motion
COPD	Chronic Obstructive Pulmonary Disease		Rx	Treatment
			$\overline{s}$	Without
CP	Chest Pain		S/Sx	Signs / Symptoms
CPR	Cardiopulmonary Resuscitation		SAMPLE	Symptoms
CSM	Circulation, Sensation, Motor Function			Allergies
CVA	Cerebrovascular Accident			Medications
d/c	Disconnect alt: Discontinue			Pertinent History
Dx	Diagnosis			Last Intake / Output
EMS	Emergency Medical Services			Events surrounding the injury
Fx	Fracture		SL	Sublingual
GI	Gastrointestinal		SOAP	Subjective information: what
GU	Genitourinary			did the pt. / bystanders say
HA	Headache			and SAMPLE
HACE	High Altitude Cerebral Edema			Objective info: Exam / Vitals
HAPE	High Altitude Pulmonary Edema			Assessment: Problem List
HIV	Human Immunodeficiency Virus			Plan: Treatment
HBV	Hepatitis B Virus		SOB	Shortness Of Breath
HTN	Hypertension		SQ	Subcutaneous
Hx	History		Sz	Seizure
ICP	Intracranial Pressure		TB	Tuberculosis
IM	Intramuscular		TBSA	Total Body Surface Area
IO	Intraosseous		TIP	Traction Into Position
IV	Intravenous		URI	Upper Respiratory Infection
kg	Kilogram		UTA	Unable to Assess
km	Kilometer		UTI	Urinary Tract Infection
LOC	Loss (alt. Level) Of Consciousness		VS	Vital Signs
mg	Milligram			P: Pulse
MI	Myocardial Infarction			R: Respirations
min	Minute			BP: Blood Pressure
ml	Milliliter			S: Skin
MOI	Mechanism Of Injury			T: Temperature
NKDA	No Known Drug Allergies			AVPU: Level of Consciousness
NVD	Nausea, Vomiting, Diarrhea		WBA	Weight Bearing Ability
O2	Oxygen		WMA	Wilderness Medical Associates
OTC	Over The Counter		y/o	Years old
$\overline{p}$	After		2°	Secondary to...(as a result of)

Read Me First

Please read the following before using the workbook

WHAT you have here is a collection of real stories gathered from Wilderness Medical Associates' Instructors. What never ceases to amaze me is the wide range of field experience distributed throughout this diverse group of individuals. As our instructors continue their involvement in patient care and the outdoors, new stories will undoubtedly filter in and it's our intention to continue to add them to the compilation you have here.

DO these patient exercises along with your Wilderness Medical Associates' courses or on your own as a review of the mental gymnastics that effective patient assessment requires. Use the sample at the front of this workbook as a reference and realize that there are a thousand ways to write this stuff down and organize your mental process. Your notes will NOT be identical to the authors but should reflect similar assessment and treatment priorities.

YOU will likely wish you had more information to supplement each of these stories especially details such as: distance to evacuation, weather, group size, etc. Including all of those details would have required a very thick book and I suspect that no matter how much background is provided, you will naturally wish for more information, as you all know..."you really had to be there". I've included what I hope will be the minimum amount of information required to make each of these a useful exercise.

THINK especially about the assessment and plan sections of the SOAP notes (the A, A',and P), but go ahead and fill in all the information on the top of the form as well (the S, and O) to get comfortable with the SOAP note format provided in the supplemental SOAP Note Book that accompanies this Workbook.

YOU WOULD be surprised to find how different the format for recording this information is from agency to agency. On the ambulance we call it a "run sheet", at the ski area, an "incident report form", in the hospital, a "chart". In our courses we call it a "SOAP note". The important thing is that the process of gathering and writing down the information is comprehensive and leaves few questions unanswered. Complete the "Questions" at the bottom of each story after you've completed your SOAP note but before you check the answers in the back of the book.

DO your best with each of these patients. Some will be very challenging when it comes to developing an assessment. You may have a hard time putting a name on things or ordering your priorities. Others are so easy you may wonder why you're doing them. These are likely the more common scenarios for us to encounter in the backcountry and are therefore worth our attention. No matter how simple or complex, each is included to make an important point. Remember the "big picture" and have fun with the stories.

Sample

The story:

A 54y/o male fell while descending a ridge on a peak in New Mexico. The route was considered 4th class and was a popular way to get up and down the mountain. The pt. lost his footing and tumbled down a steep snow slope, gaining speed, before cartwheeling into a rocky area at the base. The pt. was able to crawl to an overlook over the descent trail and call to another group for help. This group was 1000' (300m) below the pt. and began their 5 mile (8 km) descent to a National Park Service ranger station to seek help. Rescuers arrived 3 hrs. after the fall to find their pt. lying on his right side, alert and oriented, c/o severe pain in his right thigh, and pain in his right wrist. He stated he was allergic to morphine, took ibuprofen for chronic knee pain, had no other pertinent medical history, had some food and water 2 hrs. previously with his last urine output at that time, and remembered the fall vividly, denying a loss of consciousness. The pt. stated he was wearing a helmet at the time of the fall. On exam, the pt. was non-tender to the head, neck, chest, abdomen, pelvis, and spine. The pt. had some significant bruising, swelling, and was very tender on the right thigh with significantly reduced range of motion due to the pain. Swelling and tenderness was noted in the right wrist with normal range of motion and although somewhat painful, the pt. was able to flex and extend against resistance. Vitals at 1600hrs. were: Pulse: 76, Resp.: 16, B/P: 134/82, Skin: warm and normal in color, Pt. was AOx4.

Put the appropriate information from the story above into the correct spaces provided in the SOAP note to the right.

After you've completed the Subjective and Objective sections, develop an Assessment for 1600hrs. with Anticipated Problems and an appropriate Treatment Plan listed in the columns to the right.

Vitals were repeated at 1630hrs.: Pulse: 80, Resp.: 16, B/P: 128/78, Skin: normal, Pt. was Alert and Oriented and uncomfortable from the pain in his leg. No new exam findings were noted as the pt. was prepared for evacuation. Evacuation by NPS helicopter was completed at 1700hrs: Pulse: 72, Resp.: 14, B/P: 130/p, Skin: normal, Pt. is Alert and Oriented.

Put the appropriate information from the story above into the correct spaces provided in the SOAP note to the right.

Question:

1. Based on the information you have through 1700hrs., do you think this patient is stable or critical ?

* Answers to questions featured here are not provided in the "Answers" section on the back of each story, but are meant to inspire discussion with your instructor and fellow students.

SOAP NOTE

SCENE

54 y/o male fell a considerable distance down a snowfield impacting in the rocks at the base of the slope. Pt. was wearing a helmet at time of the fall and was found on his right side in the rocks 1000' (300m) above the descent trail, ~2hrs. hike from ranger station.

SUBJECTIVE

S	Symptoms	A	Allergies	*morphine*
	c/o severe pain in R thigh & some pain in R wrist	M	Medications	*ibuprofen (for chronic knee pain)*
		P	Pertinent History	*n/a*
		L	Last Input/Output	*both 2 hrs. ago*
		E	Events	*pt. denied LOC w/clear recall of events*

OBJECTIVE

Exam: *1600 hrs : Pt. Alert & Oriented. Pt. non-tender to head, neck, chest, abdomen, pelvis and spine. Bruising, swelling and tenderness noted in right mid-thigh with positive distal circulation, sensation, and a limited range of motion due to pain. Swelling and tenderness was noted in the right wrist with positive distal CSM.*

Vital Signs

Time	Pulse	Resp.	B/P	Skin	Temp.	AVPU
1600	*76*	*16*	*134/82*	*normal*	*UTA*	*Alert*
1630	*80*	*16*	*128/78*	*normal*	*UTA*	*Alert*
1700	*72*	*14*	*130/ p*	*normal*	*UTA*	*Alert*

ASSESSMENT AND PLAN

A = Assessment	A' = Anticipated Problems	P = Treatment Plan
1600 hrs:		
Unable to clear spine 2* distracting injury	*swelling / cord injury*	*stabilize / immobilize*
Unstable R upper leg injury	*swelling / ↓CSM*	*splint / monitor*
Stable R wrist injury	*swelling*	*sling & swathe / RICE*

Notes: *Pt. remained uncomfortable from the pain of his injuries, but with stable vitals throughout the course of his evacuation by NPS helicopter.*

S

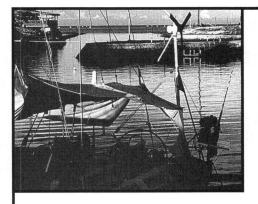

1 - FALL ON BOARD SHIP
Nova Scotia

The story:

     A 40 year old female tripped while descending a companionway amidships of a sailboat. Witnesses reported that she landed on her back on a salon table at the base of the stair, rolled onto the floor, and was found gasping for breath. As her companions started their assessment at 1100, the pts. respiratory distress quickly improved and the pt. stated that she had the wind knocked out of her in the fall. The patient complained of lower back pain but had no other complaints. She stated that she remembered tripping and falling and did not think she hit her head or neck. She had tenderness in the left flank but no bruising was noted. The abdomen was found to be soft and non-tender. The spine exam was unremarkable and she had normal CSM in all four extremities. She had no allergies, took no regular medications, and had breakfast that morning about 3 hrs. prior to the fall. Her Pulse: 98, Respirations: 22 and easy, B/P: 122/78, Skin: pale, and she was alert and anxious.

Put the appropriate information from the story above into the correct spaces provided in the SOAP note to the right.

After you've completed the Subjective and Objective sections, develop an Assessment for 1100hrs. with Anticipated Problems and an appropriate Treatment Plan listed in the columns to the right.

     At 1130, the pt. reported that her pain had diminished somewhat although a repeat exam revealed persistent left flank tenderness with some developing bruising. Her abdomen remained soft and non-tender. Vitals were repeated: Pulse 72, Skin: warm and normal in color, Respirations 14, B/P: 116/76, and her AVPU: AOx4.

Again, transfer any appropriate information to the SOAP note and update the Assessment as needed. Be sure to note the time when you update any information.

Questions:

1. Do you feel more or less comfortable with your patient at 1130?

2. If the patient did suffer significant internal bleeding from her kidney injury, what early signs might you notice during your assessment?

3. If evacuation to shore was delayed for days, what options might you have for dealing with you patients' potential spine injuy?

Assessment and Plan

A	A'	P
1100 Left flank tenderness	volume shock	PROP / monitor / EVAC
Unable to clear spine 2* distracting injury	swelling	stabilize
ASR	cont. ASR	reassurance
1130 Left flank bruising / tenderness	volume shock	PROP / monitor /EVAC

Notes:

@ 1130: ASR had resolved and vitals had improved markedly. Although the pt. continued to complain of significant pain in the left flank she was considered reliable and the spine was cleared with non-distracting off mid-line flank px and normal motor / sensory exam.

What actually happened next...

The pt. remained stable through the 8 hr. evacuation to shore and the nearest hospital. She was observed overnight and released the following day with a Dx of kidney contusion. The pt. did not sustain any other significant injury but was sore for days following the incident.

1

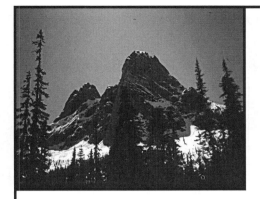

2 - FALL, GLISSADING
California

The story:

        A 2 person climbing team had just completed the North Ridge Route on the mountain and were descending the back side when they encountered a late season snowfield and opted to save time by glissading. The steep snow filled gully proved to be much firmer than anticipated and caused one of the climbers to lose control approximately 200'(60m) above the bottom of the slope. The sliding climber gained speed, bouncing off the rock walls of a constriction in the gully and continued into the talus beyond. Another party descending in the same area heard about the accident and quickly hiked the 8 miles(13km) to the trail head to notify the county sheriff. @ 1600 the pts. partner downclimbed to find his buddy awake and in severe pain from a left knee injury which was bleeding heavily. The climber wrapped his t-shirt around the pts. knee to stop the bleeding and carved out a small flat area in the base of the gully for his partner to curl up on. @ 2100, just before dark, a rescuer was flown to an LZ approx. 500'(150m) above the pt. and descended to find the patient awake and complaining of pain in his left knee, and the left side of his chest The patient had positioned himself on his left side to stabilize his injuries. The pt. & witness denied a loss of consciousness or trauma to the head and stated that the pt. was wearing a helmet at the time of the fall. The 34 y/o male pt. had some difficulty taking a deep breath when examined and was very tender to the left lateral chest with crepitus noted. Lacking a stethoscope, lung sounds were not auscultated. The pt. had sustained an extremely tender open injury to the distal left femur which bled profusely when the t-shirt was removed for examination. The pt. had good circulation distal to the injury though ROM was significantly impaired. The left arm was bruised and abraded but not significantly tender to palpation. The pts. spinal column was non-tender. The vitals were as follows: Respirations: 18, B/P: 132/p, Pulse: 76, Skin: warm, normal color, Pt. awake and uncomfortable.

Put the appropriate information from the story above into the correct spaces in the SOAP note.

Develop an Assessment for 2100hrs. with Anticipated Problems and an appropriate Treatment Plan .

    The situation necessitated a night out in the gully with a helicopter evacuation scheduled at first light. Bleeding in the knee was easily controlled with direct pressure, a splint was built and the pt. was kept as warm as possible overnight with vitals monitored periodically. @ 0500: P: 92, Skin: pale, cool, Resp.: 24 w/worsening distress, B/P: 124/p, Pt. was awake and concerned about his worsening distress.

Develop an Assessment for 0500hrs. How has your assessment changed ?

Questions:

1. On the morning of 2nd day, how worried are you about the status of this patient? Why?

2. Althought the delay in evacuation is frustrating, it allows you ample opportunity to assess and treat this patient. How might you improvise some of the treatment plan?

2

Assessment and Plan

A	A'	P
2100		
Blunt trauma to L lat. chest w/rib fx and resp. distress	resp. distress / vol. shock	PROP / monitor / EVAC
Bleeding, unstable L knee inj.	cont. bleeding / swelling	direct pressure /clean , dress / splint / monitor
Unable to clear spine 2* distracting injury	swelling	stabilize
Stable L arm injury	swelling	RICE
0500		
Comp. Volume Shock/ ↑resp. distress 2° blunt chest trauma	decomp. volume shock/ ↑respiratory distress	PROP / monitor / EVAC
Unstable L knee	swelling / infection	monitor CSM
Unable to clear spine 2* distracting injury	swelling	immobilize for transport

Notes:

What actually happened next...

The pt. continued to complain of increasing respiratory distress while the evacuation was delayed due to wind conditions. At 1400 on the 2nd day the pt. was winched aboard a hovering helicopter and flown directly to the hospital. The pt. had multiple rib fractures on the L lat. chest. A chest tube was immediately placed and approx. 1500cc of fluid was drained from the pts. chest. X-ray revealed that the pt. had sustained fractures to his distal L femur and went to surgery for repair. The pts. spine was uninjured.

2

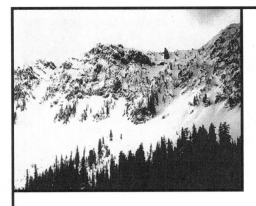

3 - SKIER HITS TREES
Alberta

The story:

     A 22 y/o female skier lost control and fell on a long, steep, icy section of a ski run. According to witnesses, she slid about 200 feet(60m) on the main run and then into the trees at a high rate of speed. At 1120hrs., ski patrolmen arrived to find the patient awake and in extreme pain, stating she impacted on her right side while sliding sideways. She was not wearing a helmet but denied hitting her head. The patient was gasping for air and complaining of severe pain to her lower back, pelvis and arm. She was only able to speak a few words at a time due to the pain she was experiencing but stated she was allergic to aspirin, took birth control pills, had breakfast about 8 that morning, and doesn't think she blacked out. On exam, she was very tender in the pelvis and lumbar spine. She had good motor and sensory function in all 4 extremities. Also noted was an angulated fracture of her right mid-shaft humerus with good distal CSM. Her vitals at 1125 were: Resp.: 28, Pulse: 116, B/P: 125/90, Skin: pale and cool, Pt. was awake and in pain.

Put the appropriate information from the story above into the correct spaces in the SOAP note.

Develop an Assessment for 1125hrs. with Anticipated Problems and an appropriate Treatment Plan .

     During transport down the mountain on a snowcat, the pt. complained of numbness in her legs and became unable to move her feet. Her vital signs @1150 were reassessed as follows: Resp.: 36, Pulse: 132, B/P: 120/88, Skin: pale, cool, clammy, Pt. was awake and very anxious.

Develop an Assessment for 1150hrs. with Anticipated Problems and an appropriate Treatment Plan .

How has your assessment changed ?

Questions:

1. A competent assessment can rule out injuries and guide the care provider in prioritizing problems. Using a risk vs. benefit analysis, can you describe any particular treatment & evacuation challenges for this patient given her injuries in this environment?

2. How might you change your perspective on these challenges if this incident occurred in the backcountry rather than a ski area?

Assessment and Plan

A	A′	P
1125 Unstable pelvic injury	volume shock	immobilize / evac.
Spine injury	swelling	immobilize / monitor
Angulated R humerus Fx	distal ischemia	TIP / splint / monitor
1150 Compensated vol. shock 2° pelvic injury	decomp. volume shock	EVAC. to ALS
Spine Injury with neuro. deficit in lower extremities	swelling	maint. immobilization and monitor

Notes:
   A neuro. deficit was noted @ 1150. Circulation remained in the lower extremities though the pt. was no longer able to feel sharp or dull sensations or move her legs.

What actually happened next...

The pt. was evacuated to the base of the ski area where a rendezvous with ALS was made. While the pt. presented with neuro. deficits in the lower extremities for some time, she suffered no permanent spinal cord injury. Her injuries included : 2 fractured lumbar vertebrae, a fractured pelvis, and a fractured upper right arm.

3

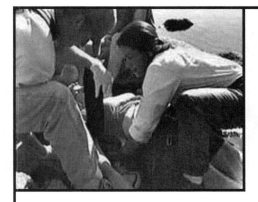

4 - FALL FROM HORSE
North Dakota

The story:

      A 45y/o female was thrown off her horse when a second horse, following too closely behind, spooked her animal. When the other riders arrived the woman was lying on her right side and not moving. Her saddle was on the ground nearby. The riders found the patient awake and anxious, complaining of pain to the right side of her chest and an abrasion to her right elbow. Pt. denied any neck or back pain. On exam @ 1500, the patient stated she had difficulty taking a deep breath, her right lateral chest was generally tender, no crepitus was noted, and lung sounds were clear and equal bilaterally. The pt. had a large abrasion to her right elbow. She was non-tender to the full length of the spine. Vitals were: Pulse: 96, Resp.: 24, B/P: UTA, Skin: pale, cool, Pt.: awake and anxious.

Put the appropriate information from the story above into the correct spaces in the SOAP note.

Develop an Assessment for 1500hrs. with Anticipated Problems and an appropriate Treatment Plan .

    Although the pt. continued to complain of pain on deep inspiration, her chest appeared on exam to be less tender and lung sounds remained clear bilaterally. Her vital signs at 1530 were: Pulse: 64R, Resp. 12 with pain on deep inspiration, B/P: UTA, Skin: warm and dry, Pt. was AOx4.

Develop an Assessment for 1530hrs. with Anticipated Problems and an appropriate Treatment Plan .

How has your assessment changed ?

Questions:

1. As the patients' ASR and Chest Wall injury appear to resolve, how might that effect your assessment and treatment plan?

2. What practical implications might your assessment have on evacuation by horseback?

4

Assessment and Plan

A	A'	P
1500		
Blunt chest trauma w/pain on deep inspiration	resp. distress / volume shock	PROP / monitor
Unable to clear spine 2* ASR	swelling	stabilize
ASR	cont. ASR	reassurance
Abrasion to rt. elbow	infection	clean and dress
1530		
Stable R lat. chest wall injury	resp. distress / volume shock	position of comfort / EVAC

Notes:

ASR resolved with time and reassurance. The elbow injury was cleaned, dressed, and bandaged and the decision was made by the group to evacuate the pt. after the spine was cleared with no tenderness to the mid-line and normal motor / sensory exam.

What actually happened next...

The pt. was evacuated by horseback without significant change in her condition. The results of evaluation in the hospital are unknown.

4

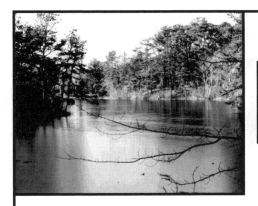

5 - DISTRESS, PORTAGING
Minnesota

The story:

A group of canoeists on a 4 day trip through the Boundary Waters stopped during a portage, when a 17 y/o male complained of difficulty breathing while lugging a canoe and oversized dry bags over the difficult terrain between lakes. The rest of the party took a break while two of the group leaders assessed the young man. At 1000hrs., the pt., complained that his chest felt "tight". He was able to speak 3-4 words at a time but stated he felt he was unable to catch his breath. The pt. stated he had no allergies, used an albuterol inhaler as needed but did not bring it with him on the trip, had a long term history of asthma, and stated that his breathing got progressively worse during the portage, until he had to stop. Vitals were: Pulse: 108, Resp.: 32, Skin: warm and sweaty, Pt. was alert and very anxious.

Put the appropriate information from the story above into the correct spaces in the SOAP note.

Develop an Assessment for 1000hrs. with Anticipated Problems and an appropriate Treatment Plan .

At 1015hrs., after rest and calm reassurance, the group leaders were able to encourage the pt. to slow and deepen his breathing. The group leaders determined that the pt. rarely suffers from asthma, and last suffered a significant attack a year prior while exercising in the cold. A repeat set of vitals were obtained: Pulse: 84, Resp. 18, Skin: warm and dry, Pt. was alert with resolving anxiety.

Put the appropriate information from the story above into the correct spaces in the SOAP note.

How has your assessment changed?

Questions:

1. If the patient did not respond to reassurance and had worsening respiratory distress, how might this episode have been managed if the group had appropriate medications?

2. Understanding the mechanism and presentation of asthma is as important as preparation with treatment options, do you fully understand the Asthma Protocol?

Assessment and Plan

A	A'	P
1000 Exercise induced asthma	↑resp. distress	rest / reassurance coach breathing
1015 Resolving asthma	recurrence	monitor

Notes:

What actually happened next...

5 The pt. was encouraged to take rest breaks and carry smaller loads during portages and continued the canoe trip without incident or recurrence.

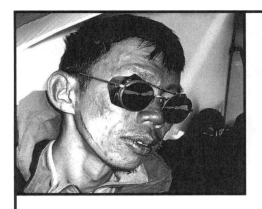

6 - BURNS, COOKING
Argentina

The story:

A pair of climbers in camp at 16,000'(4,900m) in the Andes were priming their gas stove when a fitting came loose on the fuel line and caused the stove to explode, spaying fuel over the climbers and their equipment. The tent quickly ignited and collapsed as the two climbers scrambled to escape the melting plastic. The flaming tent burned itself out rapidly and the climbers received burns of very short duration. The pt.; a 35 y/o male; who was working with the stove when it exploded complained of pain on his face. The pt. denied any allergies, was taking Diamox for altitude adaption, and was well hydrated and fueled. On exam at 1430, the pt. had already developed some redness of the forehead, nose, cheeks, chin, and on the upper neck. The nares were singed as were the hairs of the pts. mustache. The lips and the roof of the mouth appeared to be involved as well. Vitals @ 1430hrs. were: Pulse: 84, Resp.: 20 without distress, Skin: normal, Pt. was alert.

Put the appropriate information from the story above into the correct spaces in the SOAP note.

Develop an Assessment for 1430hrs. with Anticipated Problems and an appropriate Treatment Plan. What is your most significant anticipated concern ?

That night the pt. had developed some clear fluid filled blisters on the roof of his mouth, lips, cheeks, and nose. The pt. complained of discomfort and some difficulty swallowing as well as hoarseness in his voice. The pair of climbers moved into an emergency tent they had planned to use for their high camp and the pt. stated that he felt ok and wanted to continue the climb as planned. Vitals at 2100hrs. were: Pulse: 80, Resp.: 18, Breath Sounds: clear in all fields, Skin: normal, Pt. was alert.

Put the appropriate information from the story above into the correct spaces in the SOAP note.

Develop an Assessment for 2100hrs. with Anticipated Problems and a Treatment Plan.

Questions:

1. The weather and location of these climbers made descending a difficult proposition. Given the general impression above, how might you plan for managing the patient in this remote location ?

2. This story highlights the concept of "ideal vs. real" when it comes to treatment and evacuation. How many different evacuation options did you come up with?

3. If your assessment revealed wheezing, would you have picked a different option?

Assessment and Plan

A	A'	P
1430 Facial burns with respiratory involvement	swelling / pain / infection	cool / clean, dry dressing pain mgmt. / monitor / consider evacuation
2100 Progressive airway swelling	resp. distress / failure	PROP / monitor
Partial thickness facial burn	swelling / pain / infection	pain mgmt. / monitor

Notes:

What actually happened next...

The pt. complained of a sore throat and raspy painful breathing during exertion for days after his injury requiring the team of climbers to delay their summit attempt. The facial burns healed well without infection. Their summit attempt was ultimately successful.

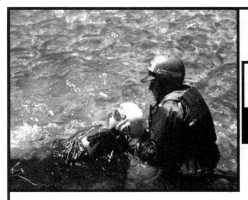

7 - FAILURE TO ROLL, KAYAK
Quebec

The story:

On a cool, rainy summer day, a 20 y/o novice kayaker flipped and failed to roll in a remote Class IV rapid in the Canadian Province of Quebec. His boat washed up in an eddy along side his floating helmet leading his rescuers to assume he had punched out and floated by. It was a couple frantic moments before the other paddlers realized that their friend was still in his kayak, trapped upside down and unresponsive. After extrication @1300, the pt. was U on AVPU and in respiratory arrest. He was quickly extricated from his boat and PPV was initiated. He still had a pulse.

Put the appropriate information from the story above into the correct spaces in the SOAP note.

Develop an Assessment for 1300hrs. with Anticipated Problems and an appropriate Treatment Plan .

After approx. 3 minutes of positive pressure ventilation, he regained consciousness and presented as awake and confused. On exam, the pt had a bruise on his L lateral forehead. His helmet had a crack through the lateral side and the chin strap was broken. There was tenderness in the lower cervical spine though no neurologic deficits were noted. The pt. was coughing intermittently and had crackles in both lower lung fields. The pt. was shivering. The rest of the exam was unremarkable. Vitals @ 1305 were: Pulse: 90, Resp.: 22 with occasional coughing, B/P: UTA, Skin: pale, cool, and wet, Temp.: UTA, Pt. was awake and confused.

Develop an Assessment for 1305hrs. with Anticipated Problems and an appropriate Treatment Plan .

SAMPLE history was largely unremarkable though it was discovered that the pt. had flipped on an eddy line at the top of the rapid and had failed to roll upright. He likely hit his head on underwater obstructions and lost consciousness.

Questions:

1. Given the respiratory injury caused by this near drowning event, how might you expect your assessment to change if the pts. respiratory status improved ? Deteriorated ?

2. What tools would you like to have on hand to manage this patient medically if you found yourself in the position of a rescuer in these circumstances ?

3. What immobilization and evacuation materials might you have on a remote river trip such as this and how might you utilize them?

Assessment and Plan

A	A'	P
1300 Respiratory Arrest	cardiac arrest	PPV
Unable to clear spine 2* unresponsiveness	swelling	stabilize
1305 Near drowning with persistent cough / crackles	↑ distress 2° pulmonary edema	PROP / monitor / EVAC
Cervical spine injury	swelling	immobilize
TBI w/forehd. bruise	↑ ICP	monitor

Notes:

What actually happened next...

The pt. remained awake and confused with a persistent cough and bilateral crackles for the remainder of the evacuation. A cervical immobilization was improvised using a PFD. The pt. was packaged in a crude hypo. wrap and transported in a kayak used as a stabilization device. Diagnosis in the hospital revealed: Concussion, Stable Fx to C5, and Pulmonary Edema due to prolonged submersion. The pt. was admitted to the ICU for a week until respiratory complications resolved.

7

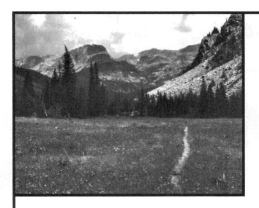

8 - FALL, MTN. BIKING
Wyoming

The story:

        A group of 4 bikers traversing a high country trail at 11,000'(3,300m) began their long descent when one of the riders missed a switchback turn and launched over his handlebars, landing on his head approx. 15'(4.5 m) over the bank. The rest of the riders found him unresponsive, his helmet cracked and called for help on a cell phone @ 1100 hrs. At 1330 the SAR team arrived after climbing 2,500'(750m) to access the patient. The pt. was found awake but subdued, oriented to person, place, time, and remembered losing control before the crash. The other riders reported the pt. had remained unresponsive for approx. 5 min. The pt. c/o a mild headache and denied vomiting, severe headache, or neck and back pain. The pt. insisted he could walk without difficulty. The pt. stated he had no allergies, took regular high BP medication, had a Hx of hypertension, had been drinking water throughout the day and had his last meal at 0800 that morning. An exam was conducted and with the exception of some minor abrasions to his arms and legs, there were no abnormalities. Vitals were: Pulse: 80, Resp.: 16, B/P: 156/100, Skin: warm and moist, Pt. was AOx4, without a complete recollection of the accident.

Put the appropriate information from the story above into the correct spaces in the SOAP note.

Develop an Assessment for 1330hrs. with Anticipated Problems and an appropriate Treatment Plan .

Questions:

1. Does a spine injury assessment and possible clearance seem appropriate to you under the circumstances ? If not, why not ?

2. How would you expect your assessment to change if the patient began presenting with increasing ICP ? Would this change your assessment if the pt. was previously cleared ?

Assessment and Plan

A	A′	P
1330 TBI	↑ ICP	monitor / EVAC

Notes:
    Spine injury R/O @ 1330 per spine assessment protocol. Pt. reliable w/o distracting injury.
Spine non-tender on exam. No deficits noted in Motor / Sensory exam.

What actually happened next...

The pt. was evacuated under his own power to the trailhead. A helicopter evac. was considered but ruled out by the difficulty of locating a suitable LZ and the patients refusal to be evacuated by air. He was transferred to the care of an ambulance crew @1700 and was seen in a hospital. He was admitted for observation and although he suffered some mild cerebral edema, a CT scan revealed no intracranial bleeding.

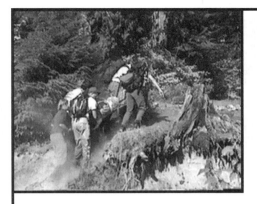

9 - FALL, HUNTING
Idaho

The story:

A man and his 18 year old son were returning from a successful goat hunt with the son carrying the goat in his pack. While descending a small talus covered ridge next to a waterfall, they separated in order to find the best way down. A short time later, the father heard a cry and the sound of rockfall. The father found his son approximately 200'(60m) down the slope at 1400hrs., unconscious, but he 'woke up' shortly after his arrival. The father made him as comfortable as possible and went for help.

What injury must you assume the son sustained given the fathers' account of the accident ?

Members of the local SAR team were notified of the accident and accompanied the father on the trip back up into the mountains. The rescuers searched all night for the injured son, locating him at first light about 650'(200m) from where his father had left him. At 0530, the pt. could not account for the events of the previous day and stated he was "a little out of it", complained of "hurting everywhere" and "being cold". The pt. c/o a headache but denied nausea or vomiting throughout the previous night. The pt. denied allergies, or regular medications, stated his last meal was a candy bar and water at 1100hrs. the previous day with last urine output some time in the middle of the night. The pt. denied a loss of consciousness and stated he was too cold and sore to sleep. The pt. was found sitting up, awake but disoriented. Exam showed small lacerations on top of his head, and chin. His right knee was swollen and tender with very little weight bearing ability. Deep lacerations to the right shin were noted. Vitals at 0530 were: B/P: 110/60, Resp.: 12, Pulse: 60, Skin: pale, cool, Temp.: 96°F (35.5°C), Pt. was Awake but disoriented.

Put the appropriate information from the story above into the correct spaces in the SOAP note.

Develop an Assessment for 0530hrs. with Anticipated Problems and an appropriate Treatment Plan.

Questions:

1. Does this patient present with signs & symptoms of increased ICP ? Are there other causes that might account for similar signs & symptoms ?

2. If a helicopter evacuation were not readily available, would you consider attempting to clear this patient of a spine injury using the Wilderness Protocol ?

Assessment and Plan

A	A′	P
1400 TBI w/significant MOI indicated by fathers Hx	↑ ICP /swelling	
0530 TBI	↑ ICP	monitor
Unable to clear spine 2* patient unreliability	swelling	stabilize
Unstable R knee injury	swelling	splint / monitor
Mild hypothermia	cont. hypothermia	dry clothes, hypo. wrap
Lacs. to R shin / head / chin	infection	clean and dress

Notes:

What actually happened next...

The patient was hoisted into a Military Helicopter within the hour after discovery by the SAR team. He suffered no lasting complications from his injuries. What happened with the goat is unknown.

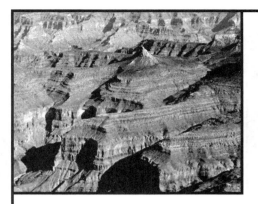

10 - FALL, SCRAMBLING
Grand Canyon

The story:

   A 32 y/o female hiking in a side canyon during a boating trip down the Colorado River fell while climbing up a loose vertical cliff band approx. 20′(6m) in height. Rescuers heard the resulting rockfall and responded to the scene within a minute of the fall to find the patient unresponsive, positioned on her side on the slope below. The pt. was found at some distance from the base of the cliff indicating she had tumbled in the fall. On exam @ 1230hrs. the Pt. was U on AVPU with rapid shallow respirations. A bleeding wound was found on the back of her head. Her clothing was torn at the shoulder and hip. Vitals were: Pulse: rapid and difficult to palpate radially, Resp.: labored, shallow, and uneven, Skin: pale, cool, clammy.

What is your immediate assessment and treatment ?

   At 1235, the patient respirations had improved, becoming more deep and even. The wound on the back of her head was found to be a 3″(7.5cm) full depth laceration at the base of her skull. Misc. bruises and abrasions were found on exam, no other obvious injuries were noted. Vitals were: Pulse: 96, Resp.: 24 and labored, B/P: UTA; radial pulses present, Pt. U on AVPU.

Put the appropriate information from the story above into the correct spaces in the SOAP note.

Develop an Assessment for 1235hrs. with Anticipated Problems and an appropriate Treatment Plan .

   Respiratory rate, rhythm, and quality continued to improve. The pt. became pain responsive, moved against attempts to stabilize her on the slope and began vomiting at approx. 5 min. intervals. At 1330, a first aid kit, backboard that had doubled as a lunch table, and other extrication gear arrived on scene from the boats at the mouth of the side canyon along the Colorado.

   The boaters were without communication in the bottom of the Grand Canyon. There were other parties on the river though their locations were unknown. Commercial parties often carry radios in this stretch of the river corridor, though they rarely work & satellite phones were then unavailable. The party has access to their 3 rafts and kayaks.

Questions:

1. What is your most important goal (and greatest challenge) in managing this patient?

2. It is easy to become overwhelmed by the risk vs. benefit decisions involved in an evacuation like this. Can you construct a rational argument for staying in place with such a patient AND an equally rational argument for evacuating this patient downriver ?

Assessment and Plan

A	A′	P
1230		
Pt. U on AVPU 2* TBI	cont.↓ AVPU/airway control	stabilize / maint. airway
Respiratory failure	respiratory arrest	PPV / monitor
Bleeding wound back of head	cont. bleeding	direct pressure / bandage
1235		
↑ICP 2° blunt head trauma w/ respiratory distress	vomiting / airway comp. resp. failure	PROP / monitor /EVAC
Unable to clear spine 2*↓ AVPU	swelling	immobilize
3″ lac. to back of head	bleeding / infection	dress / bandage
Abrasions to R hip & shoulder	infection	clean / dress

Notes:

What actually happened next...

Word of the accident passed to a second river party who pulled into the eddy at the mouth of the canyon to explore. Eventually, this party was able to pass the information on to a river trip with a radio who travelled down river to a more open area of the canyon and were able to radio relay the story to the ranger station on the South Rim.

@ 1330 The group of boaters using ropes and anchors began the evacuation of the pt. down the steep slippery drops of the side canyon moving in the direction of the river (the only practical evac. plan). During this evacuation the pt. continued vomiting at intervals and the rescuers tried to time their movements down the short vertical drops to ensure an open airway.

@ 1600 An NPS helicopter flew into the widest section of the side canyon just below the rescuers. The patient was loaded into a litter suspended below the NPS helicopter and short-hauled to an intermediate landing zone for transfer to an airmedical helicopter and a flight to the hospital in Flagstaff.

Although the pts. speech function and coordination are somewhat diminished when she is tired, she made significant neurological recovery over the course of 2 years.

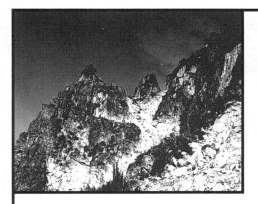

11 - FALL, TRAVERSE
Swiss Alps

The story:

A small group of mountaineers travelling just below a ridge crest were crossing a small snow field when a 23y/o male member of the group started sliding on the steep slope and quickly began tumbling out of control. The pt. travelled over 400'(120m) downhill before coming to a stop on a ledge. Rescuers arrived to find the pt. head down, unresponsive, and breathing irregularly. On exam at 1530, the rescuers discovered a large hematoma at the basilar skull with an unstable skull injury noted. An open tib./fib. fracture was noted on the right leg without active bleeding, and the pt. had sustained numerous bruises, lacerations, and abrasions. Vitals: Pulse: 124 and difficult to palpate at the carotid, Resp.: 36 and irregular, B/P: UTA, Skin: pale, cold, Pt. remained unresponsive.

Put the appropriate information from the story above into the correct spaces in the SOAP note.

Develop an Assessment for 1530hrs. with Anticipated Problems and an appropriate Treatment Plan.

The pt. was monitored closely as the group struggled to do what they could to treat the pts. injuries and initiate an evacuation plan. At 1630hrs., the pt. became pulseless and the remaining members of the group began CPR.

Put the appropriate information from the story @ 1630hrs. above into the correct spaces in the SOAP note.

Given the remote location of the group, what might be your most effective and realistic treatment plan ?

Questions:

1. In contrast to the previous incident, this story does not have a positive outcome. What do you think your greatest challenge would be as a trip leader in this situation ?

2. Once the patient lapsed into cardiac arrest, how long would you continue resuscitative efforts ? Why ?

Assessment and Plan

A	A′	P
1530		
↑ ICP 2° blunt trauma w/ unstable skull Fx	↑ ICP w/resp. compromise	PROP / monitor / EVAC
Volume shock 2* multi-trauma	decompensation	monitor / EVAC
Unable to clear spine 2* ↓ AVPU	swelling	stabilize
Open R tib. / fib. Fx	distal ischemia / infection	TIP / dress / splint
Misc. abrasions	infection	clean / dress
1630		
Cardiac arrest	cont. arrest	CPR

Notes:

What actually happened next...

Due to the difficult and dangerous access to the pt., just a couple of the party climbed down to his location and initiated care. Their initial efforts were concentrated on maintaining the pts. airway and stabilizing his position on the slope. When the pt. lapsed into cardiac arrest, the rescuers began CPR which they continued for a couple hours before deciding to stop. The pts. body was ultimately flown out by helicopter.

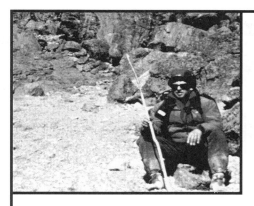

12 - FALL, DESCENDING
New York

The story:

An 18 y/o male slipped off a 12 foot(3.6 m) cliff while descending a peak in the Adirondacks. The fall was observed by the pts. partner who watched as he landed on a patch of dirt below, bounced on his side and then stood up yelling that he was ok. The pts. partner advised him not to move and the pt. complied. On climbing down to the pts. location, his partner found him breathing rapidly and complaining of pain in his left hip. The patient was sitting up, alert, and extremely anxious denying any pain in his neck or back or a loss of consciousness. The pt. stated he had an allergy to codeine, denied any regular medication, stated he had lunch at 1300. On exam @ 1500hrs., the pt. was non-tender along the spine. Chest and abdomen were non-tender. Pelvis was stable and non-tender with an abrasion noted on the left posterior hip. CSM x 4 extremities. Vitals were: Resp.: 24, Pulse: 100, B/P: UTA, Skin: pale, cool, clammy, Pt. was alert and anxious.

Put the appropriate information from the story above into the correct spaces in the SOAP note.

Develop an Assessment for 1500hrs. with Anticipated Problems and an appropriate Treatment Plan .

At 1545, the pt. had calmed considerably. Another exam was conducted without new findings. Pulse: 80, Resp.:16, Skin: normal, Pt. was AOx4.

What additional assessment might be conducted at this time ? How would you note it on a SOAP note ?

Questions:

1. **Do you think the patient sustained a positive mechanism of spine injury ?**

2. **Why did the care provider wait until 1545 before clearing the patient of a spine injury ?**

Assessment and Plan

A	A'	P
1500		
Unable to clear spine 2* ASR	swelling	stabilize
ASR	cont. ASR	reassurance
Abrasion to L post. hip	infection	clean and dress
1545		
Spine clear of significant injury (see notes)		hike out

Notes:

Spine clear of significant injury @ 1545 per spine assessment protocol. Pt. AOx4 w/o distracting injury. Spine non-tender on exam. No deficits noted in Motor / Sensory exam.

What actually happened next...

The only difficulty during the hike out stemmed from the fact that the pt. had horrible vision and had broken his glasses in the fall. Nonetheless, the pt. walked out to the trailhead by nightfall and was evaluated in the emergency dept. without findings.

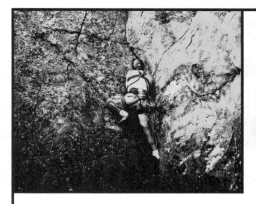

13 - FALL, ROCK CLIMBING
West Virginia

The story:

        A 40 y/o male fell while climbing at New River Gorge when his single piece of protection pulled out and precipitated a 50'(15m) fall to the ground. The pt. was wearing a helmet and a small pack. After landing on his back, he rolled onto his belly and dragged himself a short distance. One of his climbing partners reported the incident to rescuers conducting a Wilderness First Responder class nearby. At 0910, the pt. c/o pain in his legs. Pt. denied hitting his head or a loss of consciousness. On exam, the pt. was AOx4 and responding appropriately. Cervical spine was non-tender. Pt. was very tender in the lower thoracic spine with pain and tingling in both lower extremities. Pt. had a small laceration on his right forearm. The rest of the exam was unremarkable. The pt. stated he had no allergies, took no regular medications, had no previous history of back injury, had breakfast at 0700hrs. and estimated his fall distance at approx. 50'(15m). Vitals at 0910 were: Pulse: 72, Respirations: 16 without apparent distress, B/P: UTA, Skin: normal.

Put the appropriate information from the story above into the correct spaces in the SOAP note.

Develop an Assessment for 0910hrs. with Anticipated Problems and an appropriate Treatment Plan .

    An ALS ground unit was notified of the accident by phone and additional rescuers arrived to assist the original hasty team. There were no new findings during a second exam. A Motor / Sensory exam confirmed a neuro. deficit in the lower extremities (tingling). The pt. was located approx. 1 hr. by litter carry from the trailhead and from there approx. 2 hrs. by rough road to the nearest small hospital.

What might your evacuation plan be given what you know about the situation ?

Questions:

1. When patients are routinely stabilized as a precaution based on MOI alone, care providers often decide not to complete thorough spine assessments. Why should you use the Spine Assessment Protocol on a patient such as this even when he is obviously injured ?

2. How might this information effect his treatment ?

Assessment and Plan

<u>A</u>	<u>A'</u>	<u>P</u>
0910 Thoracic spine injury w/pain, tingling in lower ext.	swelling	immobilize / monitor / EVAC
Rt. forearm laceration	infection	clean and dress

Notes:

What actually happened next...

@1000 an ALS team arrived and began an IV through which they were able to administer morphine for pain. The patient was immobilized in a litter and the WFR class had the unique experience of conducting an evacuation to the trailhead. The pt. was transferred to an ambulance and driven to a landing zone where he was flown to a hospital. Follow up by local EMS representatives indicated that the pt. had indeed sustained fractures to T-12, L-1, and L-5. Bone fragments were removed during surgery and the prognosis was guardedly optimistic.

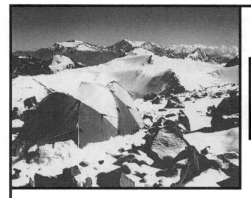

14 - AVALANCHE, CLIMBING
Washington

The story:

    A pair of friends were climbing up a steep mountain slope on a sunny spring day when the slope above them avalanched and swept the two down the mountain. After travelling approx. 1,500'(450m) in the slide, one of the climbers found himself on the surface having dislocated his shoulder in the fall. The other climber was found by his partner buried in avalanche debris up to his mid-chest and complaining of pain in his neck stating that he thought he had broken it in the fall. His partner laboriously dug him out of the debris with his usable arm and made him as comfortable as possible before descending on a 3 hr. hike out to get help from a remote townsite. Word of the accident was passed via radio and reported as a probable fatality before a rescuer arrived at 1600hrs. to find the pt. awake, disoriented, and in pain complaining that he was sure he had broken his neck. Exam showed the pts. head rotated to the right and flexed forward. Pain and tenderness in the upper cervical spine was noted and the pts. head was carefully realigned and immobilized. The pt. had a number of lacerations without active bleeding, the most significant of which was noted on the lateral aspect of the left upper leg. The patient had good circulation, sensation, and motor function in all 4 extremities. The rest of the exam was unremarkable. Vitals: Pulse: 96, Resp.: 24 and easy, B/P: 134/82, Skin: pale and cool, Pt. was awake and in pain. The pt. stated he had no known allergies, took ibuprofen for joint aches, had been well hydrated and fueled prior to the incident, remembered tumbling and falling for what seemed to him a long time, and noted that he was able to move all extremities since the incident.

Put the appropriate information from the story above into the correct spaces in the SOAP note.

Develop an Assessment for 1600hrs. with Anticipated Problems and an appropriate Treatment Plan .

Given what you know about the location of the accident, consider your options for evacuation of this patient.

Questions:

1. In this story, the patients' cervical spine was re-aligned in the field prior to evacuation. What factors would persuade you to omit or discontinue your efforts at re-alignment ?

2. How might patient alignment ease or complicate your evacuation ?

Assessment and Plan

A	A'	P
1600 Cervical spine injury	swelling	immobilize / monitor / EVAC
Laceration L lateral thigh with mult. minor lacerations	infection	clean and dress

Notes:

What actually happened next...

The pt. was evacuated just after dark by military helicopter using a winch and night vision goggles and then transferred to an ambulance for transport to the hospital. The pt. suffered multiple fractures to his vertebral column including C-1 and 2 but escaped other significant injuries. A halo stabilizer was applied to the pts. skull and he remained in the ICU undergoing a number of surgeries during his rehabilitation. The pt. suffers from a decrease in his cervical range of motion but otherwise made a complete recovery.

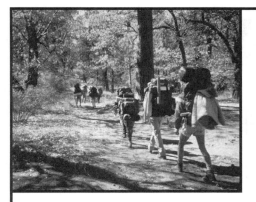

15 - SLIP, STREAM BED
New Hampshire

The story:

A group of college students was on a springtime hike along a trail in the White Mountains on a warm spring day. While crossing a small stream, a 19 y/o student slipped on wet slippery rock and fell to the stream bed. He called his companions over stating that he had injured his ankle. His fellow hikers arrived to find their friend lying in the shallow stream bed and complained of pain in his left ankle. He denied hitting his head, neck, or back. On exam at 1600hrs., the patient was awake and anxious. He was tender in his left ankle and didn't want to move it. There was no deformity, swelling, or bruising immediately evident. The patients lower extremities and clothing were wet from the fall into the shallow stream. The patient was assisted to the shore and vitals were taken: Pulse: 96, Resp.: 20, Skin: pale, cool, clammy.

Put the appropriate information from the story above into the correct spaces in the SOAP note.

Develop an Assessment for 1600hrs. with Anticipated Problems and an appropriate Treatment Plan .

What assessment criteria might be most helpful to the rescuer in determining how best to treat this injury ?

After a half an hour had passed, the pt. calmed down and was reassessed with a repeat exam revealing that the pt. could in fact move his ankle through its full range of motion although it remained "sore". There was no point tenderness noted and the pt. was able to flex and extend against resistance. Further weight bearing trials were attempted until it was determined that the pt. could bear his full weight without a pack when the ankle was wrapped with vet wrap.

Put the appropriate information from the story above into the correct spaces in the SOAP note.

Develop an Assessment for 1630hrs. with Anticipated Problems and an appropriate Treatment Plan .

Questions:

1. Which assessment criteria are most reliable and practical for determining the degree of musculoskeletal injury in these cases ?

2. What treatment strategies might be useful for "borderline" musculoskeletal injuries (those that are not OBVIOUSLY stable or unstable) ?

15

Assessment and Plan

A	A'	P
1600		
Unstable inj. to L ankle	swelling	splint and monitor
ASR	cont. ASR	reassurance
1630		
Stable inj. to L ankle	swelling	RICE and monitor

Notes:

What actually happened next...

The patients ankle was wrapped and stabilized and the pt. was evacuated under his own power to the trailhead.

15

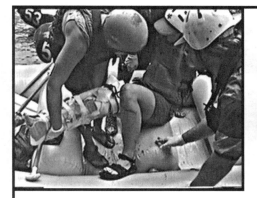

16 - WASHED OVER FALLS
Tennessee

The story:

A 25 y/o male kayaker failed to roll upright while making a move above a large waterfall and was consequently washed over the falls upside down. The crumpled kayak emerged from the hydraulic a moment later while witnesses stated it was a couple of minutes before the kayaker himself emerged from below the falls. The boater swam weakly toward an eddy below the drop while his fellow paddlers realized that the falls had ripped off his PFD, and his river shoes. At 1000hrs., the pt. stated that he thought his leg was broken. The pt. denied a loss of consciousness, or aspiration of water. On exam the pt. presented with bruises covering his body. Spine was non-tender. The pt. had a full depth laceration to his lower right leg approx. 5"(12.5cm) in length with very little bleeding. The pt. could not bear weight on the injured leg. Vitals were: Pulse: 88, Resp. 24 and easy without coughing, B/P: UTA, Skin: pale and cool, Temp.: UTA, Pt.: alert and in pain.

Put the appropriate information from the story above into the correct spaces in the SOAP note.

Develop an Assessment for 1000hrs. with Anticipated Problems and an appropriate Treatment Plan .

The wound was dressed and the pt. was warmed and reassured, calming considerably. The pt. was able to move his foot and knee through their full range of motion although painfully and was still unable to bear weight on the injured leg. Vitals were repeated at 1030 : Pulse: 80, Resp.:16 and easy without coughing, B/P: UTA, Skin: warm, Temp.: UTA, Pt. alert and calm. The paddlers found themselves on the river left bank with the only practical evacuation route lying on the opposite side. That route involved a considerable walk downstream along an old railroad grade and a difficult 4WD road to the nearest evacuation point.

Put the appropriate information from the story above into the correct spaces in the SOAP note.

Develop an Assessment for 1030hrs. with Anticipated Problems and an appropriate Treatment Plan .

What might be some evacuation options for a group of 3 paddlers in hard-shell kayaks ?

Questions:

1. Is this patients spine clearable ? If so, by what criteria ?

2. If you could not clear this patient of a spine injury, how would that effect your evacuation plan ?

Assessment and Plan

A	A'	P
1000 Unable to clear spine 2* distracting injury	swelling	stabilize
Unstable lower R leg injury w/ 5" full depth laceration	swelling / infection	clean / dress / splint / EVAC
ASR	cont. ASR	reassurance
1030 Unable to clear spine 2* distracting injury	swelling	Spine Assess. Protocol
Unstable lower R leg injury w/ 5" full depth laceration	swelling / infection	clean / dress / splint / EVAC

Notes:

What actually happened next...

The pt. was evacuated in an inflatable kayak that arrived with another group at the falls. The leg was splinted with a float bag, PFD, and throw line. The pt. was packaged in a space blanket and carried for almost 2 hrs. by paddlers using cam straps as handles on the kayak. Although the patient's leg was not ultimately fractured, he had multiple sutures to close his leg wound and did sustain injuries to several ligaments in his knee as well as a multitude of bruises.

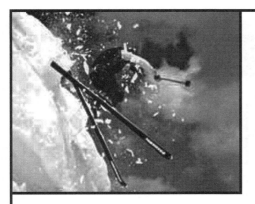

17 - FALL, OFF CORNICE
Oregon

The story:

      A 32 y/o male backcountry skiing with 3 friends, fell off a ridge when the cornice he was standing on collapsed. He tumbled approx. 150'(45m) through small trees and came to rest in a steep, narrow chute. His friends did not see the pt. fall but were able to ski down and find him within minutes. The pt. was wearing a helmet at the time of the fall. At 0700hrs., the pt. was alert and complaining of severe pain in his left hip and leg. The pt. denied a loss of consciousness. The pt. stated he had an allergy to morphine, took Ibuprofen for chronic knee pain, had breakfast at 0530, and had been keeping up with fluid intake throughout the ski trip. The pt. was extremely tender to the left pelvis and left proximal femur The left leg was externally rotated and somewhat shortened. Circulation and sensation was intact in the distal left leg and the pt. was able to wiggle his toes despite the pain in his upper thigh and pelvis. The pt. was tender to the left lateral chest wall although he was able to breathe normally, no bruising, crepitus, or deformity was noted. Minor abrasions were noted under the pts. chin where his helmet chin strap had been fastened. Vitals were: Resp.: 24, Pulse: 96, Skin: pale, cool, moist, Pt. was alert, anxious, and in pain.

Put the appropriate information from the story above into the correct spaces in the SOAP note.

Develop an Assessment for 0700hrs. with Anticipated Problems and an appropriate Treatment Plan .

      The pt. continued to complain of severe pain in his pelvis and left leg. Distal CSM remained positive in the left leg which had been splinted without traction. The pt. was immobilized as effectively as possible, packaged, and lowered down the remainder of the chute. Vitals were reassessed at 0800hrs. as follows: Pulse: 76, Resp.: 14, Skin: cool, Temp.: UTA, Pt. was AOx4 and in pain.

Has your assessment changed since 0700hrs. ?

Questions:

1. **Do you feel more or less comfortable with the patients condition after reassessment ?**

2. **What packaging techniques might be considered for a patient with injuries like these ?**

Assessment and Plan

A	A'	P
0700		
Comp. volume shock 2° unstable pelvic /femur inj.	decomp / ischemia	Immobilize / monitor / EVAC
Tenderness to L lat. chest 2° blunt trauma	vol. shock / resp. distress	PROP
Unable to clear spine 2* distracting injury	swelling	immobilize
Chin abrasions	infection	clean / dress
0800		
Unstable pelvic / femur inj.	volume shock / ischemia	Immobilize / monitor / EVAC
Tender L lat. chest	vol. shock / resp. distress	PROP
Unable to clear spine 2* distracting injury	swelling	immobilize

Notes:

What actually happened next...

The pt. was lowered out of the chute and then evacuated to an open area of level snow at the base of the slope. Eventually, the pt. was flown to a trauma center by medical helicopter, with no significant change in his condition. The diagnosis at the hospital was: 5 pelvic fractures, 3 rib fractures, and a dislocated femur. The pt. was walking unassisted 2 months later.

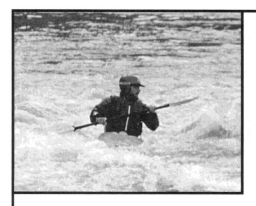

18 - WET EXIT, KAYAKING
Nepal

The story:

      A staff training group on a kayak trip was running a class III section of the river when a kayaker flipped and failed to roll. The 27 y/o male wet exited and was able to self rescue, climbing out onto a small beach bellowing in pain. At 0800, the pt. was sitting up, holding his left arm across his chest, c/o pain and immobility in his left shoulder and stated he thought he had dislocated it trying to roll upright. The pt. remembered the event, denied impact to the shoulder, head, or back and was alert and oriented. CSM X 3 with good circulation and sensation in the affected shoulder but with significantly reduced range of motion. An obvious step off deformity was noted in the left shoulder. The left humerus and clavicle were palpated without obvious instability or deformity. The pt. had sensation in the deltoid muscle of the affected shoulder. The remainder of the physical exam was unremarkable. The pt. stated he was allergic to codeine, took no regular medications, had dislocated his shoulder once before about a year previously and denied a direct impact to the shoulder. Pulse was: 88, Resp.: 20, Skin: pale, cool, Pt. was alert and in considerable pain.

Put the appropriate information from the story above into the correct spaces in the SOAP note.

Develop an Assessment for 0800hrs. with Anticipated Problems and an appropriate Treatment Plan .

Does this injury fit the guidelines of the Wilderness Protocol for Dislocation Reduction ?

      At 0830, the pt. was made as comfortable as possible and the shoulder dislocation was successfully reduced. Distal CSM was positive pre and post-reduction. The pt. was evacuated for further evaluation.

How does this treatment change your Assessment ?

Questions:

1. Does reduction of a dislocation change an unstable injury into a stable injury ? If so, how does your treatment plan change for such a patient ?

2. Do all successfully reduced simple dislocations require evacuation ? Under what circumstances might you choose not to evacuate such a patient ?

Assessment and Plan

A	A′	P
0800 L shoulder dislocation 2° indirect MOI	distal ischemia / swelling	reduce / EVAC
0830 Stable L shoulder injury (see notes)	swelling	RICE

Notes:

     Left shoulder was reduced per protocol @ 0830. Indirect dislocation with no obvious signs of fx. Pt. has Hx of previous L shoulder dislocation. Reduced with traction, abduction, and external rotation (reduced in low baseball position). +CSM post reduction. Pt. monitored during EVAC with positive distal CSM throughout.

What actually happened next...

The pt. was reduced successfully and evacuated. Distal CSM remained intact and the pt. sought further evaluation on his return to town. He continues to paddle.

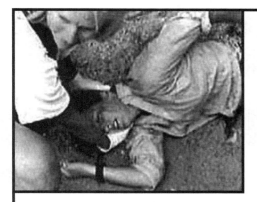

19 - NVD, HIKING
Vermont

The story:

A group of 12 young students were out on a multi-day backpacking trip in the late summer. The group travelled up a long ridge without adequate food or water and were encouraged by their trip leaders to forage for berries along the hot, steep ascent. A 15 y/o female who had been eating a variety of berries stopped after ~7 hrs. of hiking and complained of exhaustion and refused to continue. At 1500hrs., the pt. vomited several times and complained of a belly ache and exhaustion. No other observations were made by the untrained leaders of the group and no treatment was initiated, though one leader hiked out to get help.

At 2400hrs., the rescue team arrived on scene to find the pt. lying on the trail. She was incontinent of feces and urine and had obviously vomited. The shivering trip leader was found petting the pts. forehead and telling her it would be all right. All the previous pertinent medical Hx was obtained. On exam, the pt. was responsive to verbal stimulus, cool and moist to the touch, and shivering slightly. The pt. was tender to the abdomen with the rest of the exam unremarkable. Vitals were: Pulse: 112, Skin: pale, cool, moist, Resp.: 20, Temp.: 95°F(35°C) rectally, Pt. was V on AVPU.

Put the appropriate information from the story above into the correct spaces in the SOAP note.

Develop an Assessment for 2400hrs. with Anticipated Problems and an appropriate Treatment Plan .

At 0100hrs., the Pt. was cleaned up, dried off and insulated with sleeping bags in a litter. Warm IV fluids were administered and the berries the woman had been eating were identified with a description relayed by radio to Poison Control. There were now 12 rescuers on scene. Vitals were repeated: Pulse: 92, Skin: normal, Resp.: 16, Temp.: 96°F(35.5°C) rectally, although pt. had ceased shivering, Pt. was awake and lethargic.

Develop an Assessment for 0100hrs. with Anticipated Problems and an appropriate Treatment Plan .

How has your assessment changed ?

Questions:

1. It's easy to imagine the patients altered mental status being of greatest concern to you as a rescuer, what implications would this have on your evacuation plan ?

2. In the event of a long evacuation, what parameters would you monitor most closely to determine whether this patients' condition continued to improve or started to deteriorate ?

19

Assessment and Plan

A	A'	P
2400 Toxin Rxn 2° to ingestion	cont. toxin reaction	poison control / EVAC.
Comp. vol. shock 2° limited intake, sweating, vomiting, and diarrhea	decomp. shock	IV fluid replacement (if available)
Mild hypothermia	cont. hypothermia	dry clothes / hypo. wrap
0100 Mental status / vital signs improving	same as above	PO fluids as tolerated

Notes:

What actually happened next...

At 0300, Poison Control advised that although the plant was poisonous, it would generally cause symptoms no worse than vomiting and abdominal cramps. Resources were too limited to attempt a carry out over the rugged terrain that night. The pt. was monitored with a helicopter evacuation arranged at dawn. The pt. was flown to a small regional hospital where she was evaluated and transferred to a larger facility with kidney damage caused by prolonged dehydration. She spent some time in the hospital and eventually recovered.

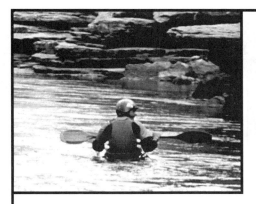

20 - STING, PADDLING
Texas

The story:

On a whitewater canoeing trip down the Rio Grande River in Texas, a 17 y/o female stepped from her boat along shore at a popular play spot. Upon exiting, she cried out and flailed her arms and legs as she jumped in the shallow water along the bank. When her fellow paddlers arrived, she stated that she was allergic to bees and she had just been stung on her right shoulder. At 1300hrs., the pt. complained of intense itchiness on her arms and legs and was extremely embarrassed to be having a reaction in front of others. The pt. stated a history of allergic reactions to bee stings, stated she has had to use an Epi-pen in the past for severe reactions but did not have her medication with her, and stated that she believed she had been stung just once on her shoulder. On exam: the pt. presented with hives on her chest, back, and face with her eyelids notably swollen. The pt. had a red swollen welt on her right posterior shoulder. Vitals were: Pulse: 100, Resp.: 30 and shallow, Skin: hives on chest, back, face, swollen eyelids, Pt. awake and anxious.

Put the appropriate information from the story above into the correct spaces in the SOAP note.

Develop an Assessment for 1300hrs. with Anticipated Problems and an appropriate Treatment Plan .

At 1315, after .3mg. of epinephrine and 100mg. Benadryl was administered, the pt. improved noticeably. The pt. stated that her face felt less swollen and skin was less itchy, though hives were still present.

At 1330, facial swelling had decreased and the pt. showed no signs of biphasic reaction. Pulse: 84, Resp.: 16 and easy, Skin: facial swelling, with some decrease in general swelling / hives, Pt. AOx4.

Put the appropriate information from the story above into the correct spaces in the SOAP note.

Develop an Assessment for 1330hrs. with Anticipated Problems and an appropriate Treatment Plan .

Question:

1. The administration of epinephrine and antihistamine for anaphylaxis is a very specific protocol requiring the care giver to understand the problem being treated, effects, side effects, dosing, route of administration and proper injection technique for these medications. Are you able to articulate this protocol in detail ?

20

Assessment and Plan

A	A′	P
1300 Anaphylaxis	resp. distress / vascular shock	.3mg epi./100mg. Benadryl
ASR	cont. ASR	treat anaphylaxis / reassure pt.
1315 Facial swelling and hives still present with improving S/Sx	cont. anaphylaxis	monitor and evac. w/ additional meds.
1330 No sign of biphasic Rxn	long term swelling	monitor and evac. w/ additional meds.

Notes:
.3mg. of epinephrine IM and 100mg. of Benadryl PO was administered @ 1305 per Protocol. Pt. has Hx allergic Rxn and presented with systemic S/Sx after bee sting. S/Sx resolved after initial dose of medications.

What actually happened next...

The patient was evacuated without rebound or incident by Wilderness First Responders for further evaluation at the hospital.

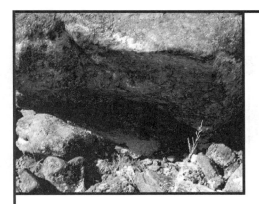

21 - SNAKE BITE, HIKING
Nevada

The story:

While hiking in a remote area of the Nevada desert, a two person party stopped for lunch in an area of large boulders in order to take advantage of the slightly cooler shady patches offered behind them. A 32yo female bent to lean her pack up against a boulder when she was struck by a rattlesnake tucked in a small hollow beneath the stone. The patient stated she heard the snake rattle just as she set the pack down but was unable to locate the source of the sound in the seconds before she was struck on the right ankle. At 1200hrs., the pt. complained of pain on her right lateral ankle calling her partners attention to 3 small puncture wounds with slight bleeding located just forward of her distal fibula. On exam: the pt. appeared to be in some discomfort, on the ground approximately 10' (3m) from the recoiled snake, holding her ankle and very anxious. The patient was assisted further away from the snake and an exam of the ankle was conducted as described above. Vitals were: Pulse: 96, Resp.: 32, Skin: slightly pale and moist, Pt. was alert and anxious.

Put the appropriate information from the story above into the correct spaces in the SOAP note.

Develop an Assessment for 1200hrs. with Anticipated Problems and an appropriate Treatment Plan .

At 1220, after her running shoe and ankle jewelery were removed for examination, the patients ankle was found to be very tender in the area of the 3 puncture wounds with an expanding area of purple discoloration around the bite. The pts. forefoot and ankle had become swollen and very painful. Pulse: 84, Resp.: 18 and easy, Skin: normal, Pt. had calmed considerably although with some evident discomfort.

Put the appropriate information from the story above into the correct spaces in the SOAP note.

Develop an Assessment for 1220hrs. with Anticipated Problems and an appropriate Treatment Plan considering that this pair of hikers is approx. 1hr. from the trailhead and then approx. 1hr. drive from the nearest paved road with an additional 1/2 hr. to the nearest hospital.

Questions:

1. Would you call this a high risk wound ? Besides the puncture wounds themselves, do you think this bite is significantly envenomated ? If so, why ?

2. What are some of your evacuation options for this patient ? How might those options affect the snake bite injury ?

Assessment and Plan

A	A′	P
1200 Snake Bite w/ high risk puncture wounds	swelling 2* envenomation / infection	clean / dress / monitor
ASR	cont. ASR	reassurance
1220 Envenomated Snake Bite	soft tissue injury / swelling / pain	splint / monitor CSM and toxin progression evacuation as tolerated

Notes:

What actually happened next...

The patient was able to hobble with significant discomfort and increasing assistance to the trailhead although it took much of the remainder of the day and the patients foot was dramatically swollen, purple, and extremely painful with progression of the swelling and discoloration to just below the knee. The patients companion transported her to the nearest hospital where she was transferred by ambulance to a larger medical center for treatment with antivenom. Her outcome is unknown.

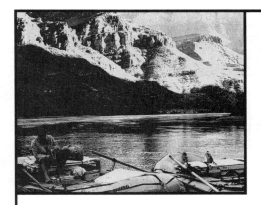

The story:

A 25y/o male raft guide on a multi-day river trip in the Southwest was stung by a scorpion while putting on river shoes he had set out the previous evening to dry. At 0830hrs., the pt. immediately hopped on one leg down to the cold river water to immerse his foot complaining of a sharp stinging pain to the arch of his right foot. The pt. stated he had no allergies, took ibuprofen for muscle aches, had no previous severe reactions to stings or bites, had eaten breakfast about an hour prior, and believed he had been stung only once. On exam, the pt. was alert and colorfully verbose, with a red marking on the arch of his right foot. He had no other complaints and pointed out the remains of the scorpion on the beach. His vitals were: Pulse: 80, Resp.: 20, Skin: pale, cool, moist, B/P: UTA.

Put the appropriate information from the story above into the correct spaces in the SOAP note.

Develop an Assessment for 0830hrs. with Anticipated Problems and an appropriate Treatment Plan .

At 0900hrs., the pt. stated that the area around the site of the sting had started to feel numb and tingling pain was now radiating up his right leg into his calf muscle. The patient stated that the cold river water did provide some relief from the pain of the sting. Although the pts. right arch had shown some swelling already, his right foot had good CSM except for a small area of numbness surrounding the site of the sting. His vitals were reassessed as follows: Pulse: 64, Resp.: 14, Skin: normal.

At 1000hrs., the group continued the river trip with another guide at the oars of the pts. boat. The swelling in the right foot had increased somewhat with numbness in most of the foot though circulation and motor function were positive. The patient began to suffer cramps in the calf muscle of the affected leg and complained of nausea.

Put the appropriate information from the story above into the correct spaces in the SOAP note.

Develop an Assessment for 1000hrs. with Anticipated Problems and an appropriate Treatment Plan.

Questions:

1. Although sharing some S/Sx with an allergic reaction, it's important to draw the distinction between this toxin exposure and an allergic reaction. What's the difference ?

2. How would you manage this patient if their symptoms progressed to facial tics and abdominal cramps ?

Assessment and Plan

A	A′	P
0830 Scorpion sting to R foot	systemic Rxn to toxin	immerse in cool water / monitor
ASR	cont. ASR	reassurance
0900 Increasing local reaction w/ numbness, swelling	pain / swelling	cont. cool water immersion / monitor
1000 Systemic symptoms	worsening reaction	OTC analgesics

Notes:

What actually happened next...

The pt. medicated himself with 100mg. of Benadryl, stating that he felt some relief from symptoms though the general feeling of discomfort continued. The patient continued to have some local cramping and numbness at the site of the sting. On the morning of the following day, the patient reported complete relief of nausea and cramping though some localized numbness remained for a number of days.

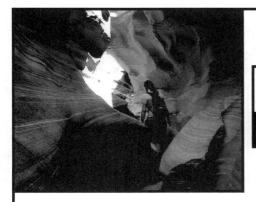

23 - BURN, CANYONEERING
Spain

The story:

A 23yo female on a remote canyoneering trip with 2 friends was boiling water for morning coffee when she knocked the pot off the rock she was cooking on and spilled much of the water onto herself. She quickly removed her boiling water soaked shorts but not before sustaining a significant burn to approximately 7% of her right thigh, crotch, and hip. Her companions immediately used a liter of treated drinking water to cool the burned area and placed the patient onto a sleeping pad to assess the injury. On exam, the pt. was alert and uncomfortable, with reddened slighly swollen skin extending from her inner thigh into the crease of her pelvis and over her right hip almost to her illiac crest. The patient suffered no burn injury to her genitals or elsewhere on her extremities. She stated an allergy to sulfa drugs and compliance with her regular medication: synthroid. Her vitals at 0730 were: Pulse: 88, Resp.: 24, Skin: normal, Pt. was alert and uncomfortable.

Put the appropriate information from the story above into the correct spaces in the SOAP note.

Develop an Assessment for 0730hrs. with Anticipated Problems and an appropriate Treatment Plan .

At 0800hrs., the group was able to acquire and treat another couple liters of potable water and further irrigated the burn, noting increased swelling and clear fluid filled blister formation beginning on the injury site. Although the patient complained of a "stinging and itching sensation", she seemed to tolerate her discomfort well. Vitals: Pulse: 76, Resp.: 16, Skin: normal, Pt. alert and somewhat more comfortable.

Put the appropriate information from the story above into the correct spaces in the SOAP note.

Develop an Assessment for 0800hrs. with Anticipated Problems and an appropriate Treatment Plan.

Questions:

1. Would you consider this burn injury to be "High Risk" ? What tools would you like to have in your first-aid kit to manage an injury like this ?

2. What implications does this injury have in the context of a Canyoneering trip where the pt. will need to negotiate technical terrain including swimming a number of pools to complete the trip or evacuate ?

23

Assessment and Plan

A	A'	P
0730 7% boiling water burn to thigh, inguinal crease, and hip	pain / swelling / infection	irrigation / dress / bandage / monitor for infection
ASR	cont. ASR	treatment / reassurance
0800 7% partial thickness burns to thigh, inguinal crease, and hip	pain / swelling /infection / function	NSAIDS / burn dressing monitor for infection / function

Notes:

What actually happened next...

The patient received 800mg. ibuprofen PO tid and her dressings were inspected 3x per day with local infection noted (pus drainage) on the end of the 2nd day. Despite efforts to reclean, dress, and protect the injury, the patient was evacuated to receive care in the hospital when her burn continued to present with persistent local infection and discomfort during travel in such a high mobility area.

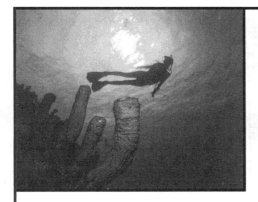

24 - BITE, SNORKELING
Florida

The story:

A couple diving off the Florida Keys split up in different directions fishing and periodically returned their catch to a boat they had anchored approx. 45 min. from the nearest port. On a return trip, the woman noticed her companion calling for help and holding his leg while swimming back to the boat. Her companion informed her that he had been bitten on his last circuit.

The pt. stated he had been bitten by a 4'(1.2m) barracuda and complained of pain in his lower right leg. The pt. stated an allergy to nuts, no regular medications, no pertinent history, stated he had last eaten at 1200hrs., and was emphatic that he was bitten once by what he could positively identify as a barracuda. On exam at 1335hrs.: the 25y/o male was in pain from the bite to his leg. The divers noted an 8"(20cm) long tearing bite wound to the pts. right anterior tibia and lateral calf muscle. The wound appeared free of major debris and bleeding was controlled effectively by a towel. Pts. Pulse: 96, Resp.: 20, Skin: pale, cool, Pt. was alert and anxious.

Put the appropriate information from the story above into the correct spaces in the SOAP note.

Develop an Assessment for 1335hrs. with Anticipated Problems and an appropriate Treatment Plan .

At 1430, the divers arrived in port for transfer to an ambulance and a 45 minute road trip to the nearest hospital. The pt. had maintained effective direct pressure on the wound during the trip to port with bleeding controlled and the pt. alert and calm.

Questions:

1. How would you realistically manage this injury if evacuation was prolonged for days ?

2. What signs and symptoms would you expect to encounter if this wound became locally infected ? How would you know the infection had become systemic ?

24

Assessment and Plan

__A__	__A'__	__P__
1335 High risk bite wound to R leg	bleeding / infection	direct pressure / thorough irrigation / dress / bandage
ASR	cont. ASR	calm pt.
1430 High risk wound	infection	EVAC. to hospital

Notes:
     The patient was an experienced diver and stated that he was positive he was bitten by a barracuda.

What actually happened next...

In the hospital it was discovered that the pts. tendon was severed in 3 places within the bite area. An extensive tendon repair was conducted as well as a debridement of the injured leg in an attempt to discourage subsequent infection. The pt. made a complete recovery and continues to thrill audiences in the pub to this day.

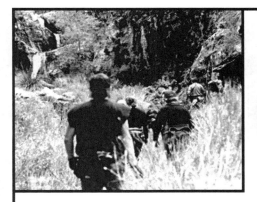

25 - BEAR ATTACK, HIKING
Montana

The story:

A hiker on a short outing from a remote trailhead was mauled by a brown bear he surprised along the way. Three other hikers discovered the pt. and sent one of their group to get help leaving the others to take care of the pt. On arrival of the rescuers at 1700hrs., the pt. stated that the bear bit him several times on the arms and then bit him on the foot pulling his boot off. He stated that he had tried to walk out but had injured himself again as he travelled barefoot down the trail. The pt. complained of pain in both arms and his right foot. He stated he had no allergies, took no regular medications, had no idea when his last tetanus shot was, had been drinking water and snacking all day, and remembered the attack in vivid detail. The pt. had 4 puncture / crush wounds of approx. 1"(2.5cm) in depth to each forearm that had resulted in some moderate blood loss but none of which was actively bleeding at the time of the exam. A 3"(7.5cm) fairly shallow laceration was noted on the bottom of the pts. right foot. The pt. had blood on his face and neck which appeared to have come from his arms as no additional wounds were noted. Pulse: 86, Resp.: 20, B/P: UTA, Skin: normal, Pt. was AOx4 and anxious.

Put the appropriate information from the story above into the correct spaces in the SOAP note.

Develop an Assessment for 1700hrs. with Anticipated Problems and an appropriate Treatment Plan .

At 1730hrs., the pts. boot was located at the mauling site a short distance back up the trail. The pt. complained of being cold and had begun shivering.

Given that the patient is approx. 2hrs. from the trailhead and then 1.5hrs. by road to the nearest clinic, what might be your evacuation plan at 1730hrs. ?

Questions:

1. Wounds such as these have a high incidence of infection and are extremely difficult to clean effectively in the field. What sort of tools would you include in a field medical kit to make that job easier and more effective ?

2. As you consider your evacuation plan at 1730hrs., can you justify a helicopter evacuation for this patient ? What if a helicopter weren't available until the following day ?

Assessment and Plan

A	A'	P
1700 High risk bite wounds to both forearms w/o active bleed.	swelling / infection	thorough PI irrigation / dress / bandage
Laceration to the R foot	infection	clean / dress / bandage
ASR	cont. ASR	calm pt.

Notes:
ASR resolved quickly with reassurance and treatment of the pts. wounds.

What actually happened next...

The pt. was evacuated to the trailhead under his own power. The pt. received a tetanus shot in the hospital and his wounds were aggressively cleaned. The pt. developed infections despite the thorough cleansing of his wounds. These were successfully treated with further wound care and antibiotics.

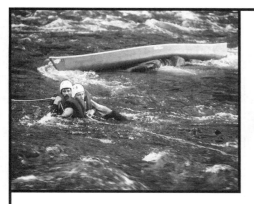

26 - BROACH, CANOEING
NW Territories

The story:

This story does not take place in a remote setting although the time interval from event to the hospital was in excess of an hour. It is included in this workbook because it is such an outstanding example and makes important points regarding both submersion and severe hypothermia.

In preparation for a canoe race, a 3-person team practiced their strokes on the river course they planned to run the following day. Spectators on a bridge over the river watched as the trio misjudged their route around a support pillar and broached their canoe on the cement piling. The bow and stern paddlers washed free of the canoe and were able to swim to shore downstream of the accident site. The pt., sitting in the center of the canoe, was pinned between the canoe and the bridge pillar as it broached and pulled underwater as it wrapped itself around the piling. Trapped between the canoe and the pillar, the pt. was submerged for 46 minutes before the efforts of rescuers resulted in her extrication. The 16y/o female was pulled from the clear 35°F(2°C)water with her lifejacket still on and moved quickly to a waiting ambulance. At 1400hrs. the pt. was pulseless and extremely cold to the touch with facial edema and peripheral cyanosis noted on exam.

Put the appropriate information from the story above into the correct spaces in the SOAP note.

Develop an Assessment for 1400hrs. with Anticipated Problems and an appropriate Treatment Plan .

At 1403hrs., the pt. was pulseless and a cardiac monitor showed fine ventricular fibrillation. The pt. had a rectal core temperature of 73°F(22°C).

What are your primary treatment concerns with a pt. like this ?

Questions:

1. How might your treatment for this pt. vary in an ambulance vs. wilderness environment ?

2. If a helicopter evacuation was available in a wilderness setting *within an hour*, would that change your treatment plan in a remote setting ?

Assessment and Plan

<u>A</u>	<u>A'</u>	<u>P</u>
1403 Cardiac arrest 2° drowning	cont. cardiac arrest	PPV / CPR ?
Severe hypothermia	cont. hypothermia	carefully handling/ ALS

What actually happened next...

In the hospital, the pt. was rewarmed 2°F(1°C)/ hr. through the use of a ventilator, warmed IV fluids, rectal lavage, peritoneal lavage, and kidney dialysis (the hospital did not then have a heart bypass system). During the rewarming period, the pt. regained a perfusing pulse and then arrested on 3 occasions. Each time the pt. was resuscitated with defibrillation and minimal dose medications. The pt. was transferred from the emergency dept. to the ICU with a gag reflex and a B/P of 90/50 which led to cautious optimism amongst care providers. Two days after the event, sedation was decreased and the pt. woke up and waved to her parents responding appropriately to simple stimulus. Two weeks after arrival the pt. was extubated and controlled her own airway effectively. After a month of intermittent setbacks, especially respiratory infections, the pt. was discharged to a rehabilitation center and continues to make improvement to this day.

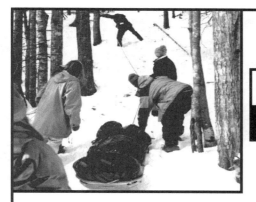

27 - WINTER BACKPACKING
Yukon

The story:

A group of 12 college students arrived at the trailhead at the end of Jan. and started up the trail in 0-10°F(-15°C) temperatures on a multi-day backpacking trip breaking trail through one and a half feet of new snow for 5 hrs. before stopping for lunch. The 19 y/o female pt. did not eat or drink at the rest stop. After lunch, the group then began their steep, 3 mile(5km) climb , passing a ranger station and arriving at camp @ 1800hrs. They had been breaking trail for approx. 10 hrs. with full packs.

The pt. was "tired" and wanted to rest before dinner. When her partner went to wake her at 2000hrs., she was very cold and would not wake. Vitals were: Pulse: 40 and regular at the carotid, Resp: 8 and shallow, B/P: UTA, no radial pulse palpable, Skin: pale, cold, Temp: 86°F(30°C) orally, Pt. was unresponsive.

Put the appropriate information from the story above into the correct spaces in the SOAP note.

Develop an Assessment for 2000hrs. with Anticipated Problems and an appropriate Treatment Plan .

3 students returned to the Ranger Station seeking help (approx. 1mile down the trail) and arrived back at the camp about 2100hrs. The caretaker of the cabin (a WEMT) arrived with a toboggan and on assessment found the patient cold, unresponsive, and cyanotic around the lips and extremities. The patients medical history was obtained from the trip leader and there were no new findings. Vitals were reassessed: Pulse: 36, Resp.: 8, B/P: UTA, Skin: pale and cold, Temp.: 88°F(31°C) rectally, Pt. was unresponsive.

At this point it started to snow and the pt. was carefully transported by toboggan back to the caretakers cabin arriving at 2300hrs.

Noting the time, distance to evacuation, and conditions on the trail, what might some of your treatment and evacuation options be ?

Questions:

1. Are there any other problems to consider in the differential diagnosis of this patient if, for instance, the rescuers lacked a suitable thermometer ?

2. If you encountered such a situation without access to a cabin and an unlimited heat source, how might you alter your treatment and evacuation plan ?

Assessment and Plan

A	A'	P
2000 Severe Hypothermia	↑ hypothermia respiratory failure	careful handling, prevent further heat loss & prep. for evac.
2100 Severe Hypothermia	↑ hypothermia respiratory failure	careful evacuation & monitoring
2300 Severe Hypothermia	↑ hypothermia	PPV / gradual rewarm./ closely monitor vitals

Notes:

As evac. was impossible given the conditions @ 2300, the decision was made to gradually rewarm the pt. by increasing the heat and humidity inside the cabin and continuing ventilations.

What actually happened next...

As careful evacuation to the trail head was next to impossible given the conditions, the caretaker slowly increased the heat and humidity in the cabin by placing water pots on the cookstove and keeping the fire stoked up. The patient remained U on AVPU. Her core temperature was taken at 86°F(30°C) and the rescuers began ventilations. After 2 hours, her core temp. rose to 90°F(32°C) though the pt. remained unresponsive. Nearly 5 additional hours of artificial ventilations and slow warming resulted in a core temp. of 94°F(34°C) and the pt. became V on AVPU. Within an hour, the patient regained consciousness and remained awake during the subsequent evacuation.

Consider the resources required for this positive outcome and the narrow window of opportunity to intervene. This is certainly an exceptional case and supports a careful case specific approach to management of the hypothermic pt.

27

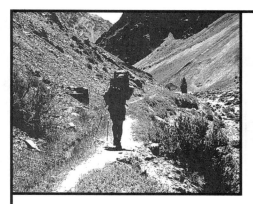

28 - EXHAUSTION, HIKING
Chile

The story:

Hikers responded to a 27 y/o male lying off the edge of the trail in the Andes. The pt. stated that he had climbed to a peak that morning and was half way back down (a vertical gain and subsequent loss of almost 8,000 feet(2,400m)) when he started to feel sick and unsteady. He was carrying a coke bottle from which he had drunk approximately 2 liters of water since his morning departure 9 hours before. Ambient temperature was 99°F(37.5°C). The pt. complained of weakness, nausea, dizziness on standing, and stated he last urinated approx. 6 hrs. previously. Pt. denied that he had blacked out at any point prior to arrival of the hikers. He stated a history of allergies to pollen for which he took antihistamines, had no other relevant medical history, stated he hadn't eaten since breakfast and had a total fluid intake of less than 2 liters of water over the course of his 9hr. climb. At 1500hrs., the pt. was lying on his side, AOx4, with pale, cool skin. Vitals taken supine: Pulse: 100, Resp.: 20, B/P: 94/50, Skin: pale and cool, Temp.: 98.5°F(37°C) orally, Pt. was AOx4. Vitals taken standing: Pulse: 124, Resp.: 24, B/P: 90/50, Skin: pale, cool, Pt. was AOx4 with increased dizziness.

Put the appropriate information from the story above into the correct spaces in the SOAP note.

Develop an Assessment for 1500hrs. with Anticipated Problems and an appropriate Treatment Plan.

Questions:

1. What are the most useful elements of the PAS for determining the problem and the most appropriate treatment ?

2. How could the patients current problem lead to heat stroke or hyponatremia if unresolved in this environment ?

Assessment and Plan

A	**A'**	**P**
1500 Heat Exhaustion (compensated volume shock 2* dehydration)	decompensation / heat stroke	gradual PO fluid & electrolyte replacement / continued VS monitoring

Notes:

The pt. was successfully rehydrated and fueled and after a long rest, completed the descent in the cooler hours of the early evening.

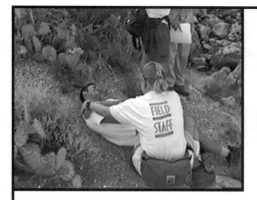

29 - SEIZURE, HIKING
Arizona

The story:

A group of hikers encountered a 51y/o male on the Bright Angel Trail in Grand Canyon. The trip leader stated that he did not think the man had any medical condition and was not taking any medication. Before collapsing, the man became disoriented and appeared to hallucinate. Moments after collapsing, the group observed muscle twitching which they described as a seizure. The trip leader stated the pt. had last eaten a couple of hours previously and he guessed his fluid intake at 2-3 liters over the course of the morning. The leader stated the group had hiked almost 10 miles(16km) over rugged terrain since their morning departure in ambient temperatures of 90°F(32°C). On exam at 1330hrs., the pt. was found supine with his eyes open, mumbling incomprehensibly. Pt. was maintaining his own airway though he did not respond to questions. Skin was very warm, moist, and flushed. Pts. clothes were soaked in sweat, and he was incontinent of stool and urine. Pulse was: 164, Resp.: 34, B/P: UTA, though strong radial pulses were present, Temp.: 107°F(41.5°C) rectally, Pt. responded to painful stimuli.

Put the appropriate information from the story above into the correct spaces in the SOAP note.

Develop an Assessment for 1330hrs. with Anticipated Problems and an appropriate Treatment Plan .

Questions:

1. **What are the most useful elements of the PAS for determining the problem and the most appropriate treatment ?**

2. **Although it's likely that you can readily identify elements of the PAS that allow you to determine the problem, what questions not included here, would yield useful information ?**

Assessment and Plan

A	A'	P
1330 Heat Stroke	seizure, death	rapid cooling / EVAC

Notes:

What actually happened next...

The pt. was cooled by being soaked with water and fanned aggressively. IV fluids were administered and the pt. was evacuated by helicopter to the hospital. The pt. survived though his disposition after treatment in the hospital is unknown.

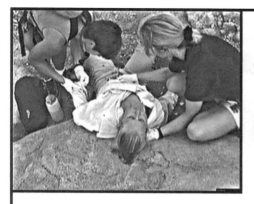

30 - CRAMPS, HIKING
Canyonlands

The story:

A 36 y/o female on her second day visiting from Europe, hiked alone from the Island in the Sky Ranger Station to an overlook above the confluence of the Colorado and Green Rivers. This arduous hike involves travel on jeep roads and rugged trails with a significant elevation loss and gain. Mountain Bikers on the White Rim Trail encountered the woman lying in the trail huddled in a ball, shaking. The pt. complained of feeling miserable: dizzy, sluggish and cold (despite the 90°F(32°C) plus temps.). The pt. stated she had been drinking water continuously during the day and experienced bouts of nausea just after leaving the overlook on her way up. The pt. c/o muscle cramps in both legs. The pt. stated she had no allergies, took no medications regularly, estimated she had urinated x 6 over the last couple of hours, denied any recent illness or infection, had eaten a rice cake with peanut butter approximately 6 hrs. previously, and estimates she has had 5 liters of water. On exam at 1645hrs., the pt. was found balled up on the trail awake and responding sluggishly to questions. She was pale and generally tremulous while a physical exam was conducted without other significant findings. Pulse: 104, Resp.: 24, B/P: 100/66, Skin: pale, cool, moist, Temp.: 96.5°F(36°C) orally, Pt. was awake and slow to respond. During an hour and a half in the care of the mt. bikers, the pt. passed urine x2 and complained of thirst.

Put the appropriate information from the story above into the correct spaces in the SOAP note.

Develop an Assessment for 1645hrs. with Anticipated Problems and an appropriate Treatment Plan .

Questions:

1. What are the most useful signs and/or symptoms for determining the problem and the most appropriate treatment ?

2. Especially with exertion in a hot environment, fluid replacement is only half the equation. What strategies might you use to prevent such problems ? How might you measure success ?

Assessment and Plan

A	A′	P
1645 Depleted electrolytes (hyponatremia)	↓AVPU / seizures	carefully replace fluids & electrolytes / EVAC

Notes:

What actually happened next...

A dilute sports drink was given in quantities sufficient for the patient to swallow small amounts of salty trail snacks as tolerated to replace electrolytes. The patient was evacuated by ground to the nearest hospital for evaluation. The pt. was diagnosed with hyponatremia (low serum sodium) which was gradually adjusted with IV normal saline. The patient spent the night in the hospital and was discharged with normal labs & without symptoms the next day.

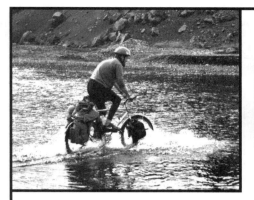

31 - WEAKNESS, BIKING
Iceland

The story:

A pair of mountain bikers exploring a remote valley in the interior of Iceland had spent a long day biking and alternately carrying their bikes through thick mud and multiple stream crossings. At 1925, the pt., a 27 y/o male complained of weakness, dizziness, and stated he was having difficulty balancing on his bike. The pt. had no allergies, took no regular medication, had last eaten at 1330 with water intake at regular intervals, and had been mountain biking since 0800 that morning. The pts. partner found him pale, sweaty, and shaking in the extremities with some obvious difficulty balancing. The pt. had no recent history of injury or illness. Pulse was: 88, Resp. 20, Skin: pale, cool, moist, Pt. was awake and lethargic in answering questions.

Put the appropriate information from the story above into the correct spaces in the SOAP note.

Develop an Assessment for 1925hrs. with Anticipated Problems and an appropriate Treatment Plan .

At 1945, after resting a few minutes, eating some carbohydrates, and hydrating, the pt. felt much better. Trembling in the extremities quickly resolved and the pt. no longer felt dizzy or weak. The pair continued their trip to camp without incident.

Questions:

1. If this pt. were a diagnosed diabetic, would this change your treatment plan ?

2. If the hypoglycemia became progressively worse for this patient, what other signs and symptoms might you expect ?

Assessment and Plan

A	A'	P
1925 hypoglycemia	↓mental status	feed and hydrate / monitor

Notes:

What actually happened next...

After further hydration and additional carbohydrates, the pt. was asymptomatic and able to continue biking without recurrence.

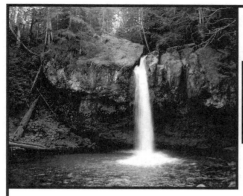

32 - SEIZURE, BACKPACKING
South Carolina

The story:

An 8 person group on a multi-day backpacking trip in the mountains was searching for a suitable campsite just before dark when at approx. 2000hrs., a 13yo male member of the party who was resting against a tree, tipped over, and began what appeared to be a full body seizure. His clonic convulsions lasted approx. 1 minute before terminating spontaneously followed by a flaccid unresponsive period. On exam: Pt. was pale and cool. Pupils were equal and reactive to light but not tracking. The rest of the physical exam was unremarkable and the patient appeared atraumatic. Pulse: 108 and regular, Resp.: 40 and shallow initially. Pt. remained unresponsive.

Put the appropriate information from the story above into the correct spaces in the SOAP note.

Develop an Assessment for 2000hrs. with Anticipated Problems and an appropriate Treatment Plan.

After an intial period of unresponsiveness lasting approx. 5 min. after the seizure, the patient gradually began some spontaneous movement of the face and extremities accompanied by moaning and response to painful stimuli. After a few more minutes the patient responded to verbal stimuli with more coordinated spontaneous movement, eye opening, and unintelligible speech. By 2030 hrs., the patient appeared exhausted but awake able to respond to simple questions in a sleepy but intelligible pattern of response denying any focal discomfort aside from being "tired". The patient denied any history of previous seizure and responded in the negative when asked if he had previous medical history of any kind. The patients pre-trip medical screening form showed no previous medical history, allergies, or regular medications.

Put the appropriate information from the story above into the correct spaces in the SOAP note.

Develop an Assessment for 2030hrs. with Anticipated Problems and an appropriate Treatment Plan.

Questions:

1. In the absence of a suggestive medical history, what factors could have caused this patient to suffer a seizure ?

2. What sorts of evacuation options would you consider with a patient such as this and what measures would you take to prevent recurrence of another seizure en route ?

Assessment and Plan

A	A'	P
2000 seizure without previous Hx / or known cause	cont. seizure activity	monitor critical systems / reassurance
2030 status post seizure, ↑ AVPU	recurrent seizure	hydrate / fuel / monitor EVAC in morning

Notes:

What actually happened next...

The pt. had just completed a fairly exhausting day on the trail and without an otherwise suggestive history was treated as dehydrated and calorie & electrolyte depleted. The patient was comfortable and seizure free throughout the night, was able to hike out under his own power in the morning, and was transported to the nearest hospital for evaluation. His evaluation in the hospital was unremarkable without a definitive diagnosis regarding the cause of the seizure.

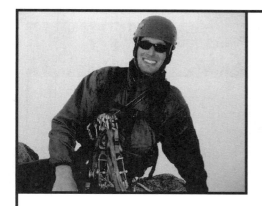

33 - ATAXIA, CLIMBING
Wyoming

The story:

A 21yo male, accompanied by two companions, completed an ascent of Exum Ridge on the Grand Teton. The small group had approached the mountain by climbing approx. 5,000' (1,500m) on the previous day to camp in preparation for the technical portion of the climb. Getting an alpine start, the group moved readily up the numerous rock pitches in fine weather to achieve the summit: 13,700' (4,200m) at approx. 1200hrs. After a short break the climbers scrambled down to the fixed anchors for the rappel to the Upper Saddle when the 21yo male complained of a headache and dizziness stating he was having trouble with his balance as he arrived at the stance. He began stacking rope for rappel and fumbled repeatedly with the knot joining two ropes before his companions noticed his error and relieved him of the rigging.

Put the appropriate information from the story above into the correct spaces in the SOAP note.

Develop an Assessment for 1200hrs. with Anticipated Problems and an appropriate Treatment Plan .

At 1230hrs., one companion preceeded the patient on the rappel leaving the other to assist him with his rigging and follow behind. The patient was able to descend to the Upper Saddle but complained his symptoms were worsening with an increasing headache, dizziness, and nausea. While the third climber completed his rappel, the patients companion completed a set of vitals: Pulse: 88, Resp.: 24 without apparent distress, Skin: slightly pale, Pt. was alert and aware of his slight disorientation. The 3 climbers continued their scramble from the Upper Saddle down towards the Lower Saddle with the patient continuing to complain of symptoms, stumbling occasionally, and suffering a single episode of vomiting just before reaching the Lower Saddle: 11,500' (3,500m) at approx. 1500hrs.

Put the appropriate information from the story above into the correct spaces in the SOAP note.

Develop an Assessment for 1500hrs. with Anticipated Problems and an appropriate Treatment Plan.

Questions:

1. If the patient had been unable to complete the rappel below the summit, what other alternatives would you consider for treatment or evacuation ?

2. If the Lower Saddle offered shelter and the possibility of a delayed helicopter evacuation (or) your party could descend in relative safety to the level of the previous nights camp and even lower below 9,000', which option would you choose and why ?

Assessment and Plan

A	A'	P
1200 headache & ataxia 2* presumed HACE	↑ ataxia, ↓ mental status	feed & hydrate / monitor / descend cautiously
1500 HACE	↑ ICP	descend & monitor

Notes:

What actually happened next...

The patient was able to descend under his own power under the watchful eyes of his companions and improved with resolving nausea, headache, and ataxia with descent below the Lower Saddle and then below 9,000' (2,700m). The patient was symptom free the following morning and completed the rest of the return trip without incident.

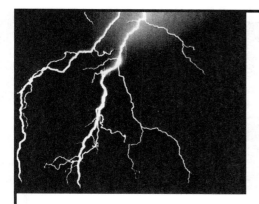

34 - LIGHTNING STRIKE
North Carolina

The story:

     A 3 person party had set up camp among the trees in the mountains. Thunderstorms had been moving through the area all day and into the evening. At approx. 2130 hrs. a lightning strike occurred nearby and one of the party sleeping in his own tent was struck. His partners reported that the 17 y/o male pt. initially presented thrashing but awake in his tent . The pt. was unable to speak, had some difficulty breathing, and all the hairs burned off of his legs. One of the backpackers hiked out 2 miles(3.2 km) to the trailhead and called for help. The rescue team arrived at 0200hrs. to find the pt. awake and in distress. The pt. primarily complained of pain in his legs where he had been burned (the tent had a distinct smell of burned hair). The pt. was able to speak at this time and stated he had no allergies, took no regular meds, had no cardiac history, had eaten dinner about 6hrs. ago, stating he did not remember being struck though his friends were sure he was. On exam: Pt. was sweaty and pale with superficial burns (looking like sunburn) to both legs. The rest of the physical exam was unremarkable. Pulse: 124 and irregular, Resp.: 28 and mildly labored, B/P: 135/p, Skin: pale and moist, Pt. awake and in distress.

Put the appropriate information from the story above into the correct spaces in the SOAP note.

Develop an Assessment for 0200hrs. with Anticipated Problems and an appropriate Treatment Plan.

Questions:

1. Despite the patients apparent "stability" on scene, what are some anticipated problems of significant concern ?

2. How might these concerns effect your evacuation plan ?

Assessment and Plan

A	**A'**	**P**
0200 Lightning strike w/cardiac and resp. abnormalities	cardiac dysrhythmias / respiratory distress	monitor / EVAC to ALS
Superficial burns to legs	pt. discomfort	sterile dressings

Notes:

What actually happened next...

The pt. was evacuated at first light by litter over a muddy mtn. trail requiring 4 hrs. to reach the trailhead. Vital signs remained relatively unchanged throughout transport. He remained in the hospital for 4 days and was released. Victims of significant lightning injury often complain of long term deficits though follow-up for this patient is unknown.

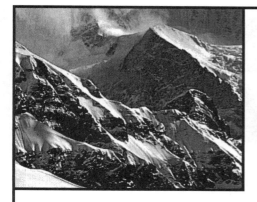

The story:

A group of climbers had achieved their goal of summiting a peak in Alaska when they noticed the weather deteriorating. They opted to continue down past their high camp hoping to descend to the 14,000'(4,200m) level before the imminent storm arrived. During the descent, the winds increased to 60 m.p.h.(97 kph) with temps. of approx. 0°F(-17°C). On arrival at the 14,000' camp, a 28 y/o female complained of painful, stiff hands. Apparently, while adjusting her crampons a couple of hours earlier, the wind had blown away her overmitts and not wishing to slow the descent, she hadn't called for a stop to replace them. At 1800hrs., the pt. stated that she thought the sensation in her fingers had been absent for a "couple of hrs". On exam, the patient was awake and in pain. The thumb, first, and second digits on her right hand were white and hard to the touch up to the second knuckle. The other two fingers were white and hard to the first knuckle. There were a couple of white patches on the right side of the pts. cheek though these were soft to the touch. Vitals: Pulse: 96, Resp.: 20, Skin: normal except as noted above. Pt. stated she had no known allergies, took Diamox 125mg. twice a day, had never sustained a frostbite injury before, had last had a cliff bar 3 hrs. previously and had not had much water since midday.

Put the appropriate information from the story above into the correct spaces in the SOAP note.

Develop an Assessment for 1800hrs. with Anticipated Problems and an appropriate Treatment Plan .

At 1700hrs. (23hrs. later), the storm had raged all night and was likely to continue through a second night making an evacuation impossible. All the climbers had spent the storm adequately sheltered in tents melting snow and rehydrating from the long summit day. The pts. fingers had been wrapped with gauze and the patchy areas of frostnip on her face had been rewarmed immediately with skin contact. She had been taking large doses of ibuprofen since her arrival in camp but the pain from her slowly rewarming digits had become almost unbearable. Already, there were blood filled blisters forming on the injured fingers.

Put the appropriate information from the story above into the correct spaces in the SOAP note.

Develop an Assessment for 1700hrs. with Anticipated Problems and an appropriate Treatment Plan .

Questions:

1. If your evacuation plan included traversing nontechnical terrain to air evacuation as soon as the storm cleared, how might this situation be managed ?

2. What about a more remote setting with technical terrain and no possibility of assisted evacuation ?

Assessment and Plan

A	A'	P
1800 Frostbite R fingers (hard)	swelling / pain w/rewarming	dress / monitor
Frostnip R cheek (soft)	frostbite	immediate rewarming hydration / food
1700 (day 2) Passively rewarming frostbitten fingers	pain / swelling / infection	change dressings pain meds / monitor

Notes:

What actually happened next...

Given that the patient could access air evacuation relatively easily, the fingers were immediately rewarmed in a pot of water kept at 105°F(41°C). Large blood filled blisters formed within 24 hrs. post rewarming and the first and second fingers turned purple. The pt. was flown from the mtn. as soon as the storm cleared and transferred to the hospital where tissue was debrided from the tips of all fingers. Nails on the thumb, first, and second fingers were lost and never grew back.

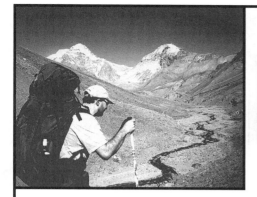

36 - DISTRESS, ALTITUDE
Bolivia

The story:

While climbing in Bolivia at 18,000'(5,500m) a 35 y/o male developed shortness of breath, weakness, and slight ataxia. The group of climbers had acclimatized at 13,000'(3,900m) for 4 days, then 15,000(4,500m) for 2 days and were going to set up a high camp with plans to return to sleep at the lower elevation that night. The group had not experienced any problems with altitude up to that point. At 1300hrs., the patient began to complain of SOB and weakness. He was having a hard time standing up straight. He denied headache or any serious neurologic complaints. The pt. stated he had no allergies, had been taking low doses of Diamox throughout the trip, had no previous difficulty at altitude, was well fueled and hydrated, and stated his symptoms had come on gradually over the last 2 hrs. The pt. had crackles in both lower lung fields when a stethoscope was used to auscultate his chest. Pulse: 116, Resp.: 30 and labored, Skin: normal, B/P: UTA, Pt. was alert and anxious.

Put the appropriate information from the story above into the correct spaces in the SOAP note.

Develop an Assessment for 1300hrs. with Anticipated Problems and an appropriate Treatment Plan .

Questions:

1. If the patient had not presented with crackles on auscultation of his chest, would that change your treatment plan ?

2. What treatment measures might you utilize if weather or environmental conditions made descent impossible ?

36

Assessment and Plan

A	A′	P
1300 Resp. distress 2* HAPE	severe HAPE	immediate descent
Ataxia	fall	assisted descent

Notes:

What actually happened next...

The pt. was assisted by team members down to the 15,000′(4572m) level with almost complete relief of symptoms. The next day the pt. felt well but slight crackles were still present in the lower lung fields so the team continued their ascent without him. Although disappointed, the patient was able to play a helpful role in assisting other ill climbers struggling with their own difficulties at altitude.

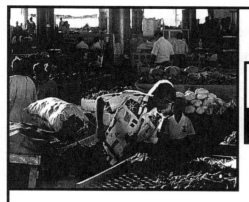

37 - GI DISTRESS, TREKKING
Mexico

The story:

      A group of international studies students stopped at a street vendor for a meal in a remote town in Mexico. Within a couple of days the whole group suffered from intestinal complaints including persistent diarrhea and vomiting. In most cases the symptoms of illness had passed within 12 hrs. One female student complained of continuing symptoms over a 3 day period.

Day 1

  The pt., a 20 y/o female complained of severe abdominal and intestinal cramps a couple hours after her last meal. Later that same day, she started to experience diarrhea and vomiting. The pt. stated she was allergic to shellfish (there was none in the suspect meal), took no regular medications, hadn't been able to keep food or fluids down since lunch 8hrs. previously. Her vitals were: Pulse: 76, Resp.: 16, B/P: UTA, Skin: warm, moist, Temp.: 97°F(36°C), Pt. was alert and uncomfortable.

Put the appropriate information from the story above into the correct spaces in the SOAP note.

Develop an Assessment for Day 1 with Anticipated Problems and an appropriate Treatment Plan .

Day 2

  The diarrhea and vomiting continued despite the pts. attempts to keep down simple foods and fluids. The pt. c/o a headache, cramps, chills, NVD, and stated she felt feverish. Her vitals on day 2: Pulse: 92, Resp.: 24, Skin: pale, cool, moist, Temp.: 103°F(39.5°C), Pt. was awake, sluggish, and uncomfortable.

Put the appropriate information from the story above into the correct spaces in the SOAP note.

Develop an Assessment for Day 2 with Anticipated Problems and an appropriate Treatment Plan .

Questions:

1. **What is your primary management problem for this patient ?**

2. **How might this patient be managed if evacuation is significantly delayed ?**

Assessment and Plan

A	A′	P
Day 1 GI infection	NVD / volume shock	replace electrolytes as tolerated / Pepto / monitor
Day 2 Systemic Infection	vascular shock	antibiotics / antipyretic
Comp. volume shock	decomp. volume shock	replace PO fluids as tolerated / EVAC

Notes:

What actually happened next...

The whole group of students suffered from this GI bug though all except this pt. recovered in a day or so. An antidiarrheal was not used by any members of the party though pepto-bismol helped with symptoms. The woman was evacuated and treated with antibiotics which were ultimately successful in treating the infection.

37

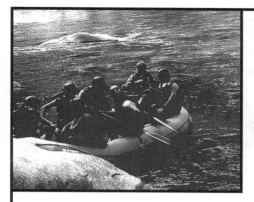

38 - ABD. PAIN, RAFTING
Colorado

The story:

A 22y/o female river guide complained to her coworkers of a gradual onset of abdominal pain over the previous 36hrs. She stated she dismissed the pain initially as an intestinal problem but became concerned as the pain intensified and her efforts to alleviate it were unsuccessful. Her coworkers took a set of vitals at 1900hrs.: Pulse: 72, Resp.: 16, Skin: normal, Pt. was alert and uncomfortable.

Put the appropriate information from the story above into the correct spaces in the SOAP note.

Develop an Assessment for 1900hrs. with Anticipated Problems and an appropriate Treatment Plan . What questions would you like to ask this pt. ?

At 2000hrs. the pain had increased, was constant, focal in the lower right quadrant, and the pt. described it as an 8/10. The pt. stated she had an allergy to penicillin, and took no regular medications. She stated she had her appendix removed when she was 15, was sexually active, used a diaphragm for birth control, had missed her last menstrual cycle which she attributed to her recent activity levels, had never been pregnant, and stated she did not think it possible presently. She was well hydrated and fueled and denied any recent GI/GU problems. Vitals at 2000hrs.: Pulse: 92, Resp.: 20, Skin: pale, cool, Temp.: UTA, Pt. was alert and stated her pain was 10/10 and guarding when her abdomen was palpated for tenderness.

Put the appropriate information from the story above into the correct spaces in the SOAP note.

Develop an Assessment for 2000hrs. with Anticipated Problems and an appropriate Treatment Plan. If you were in a location with possible satellite phone communications, how would that change your Treatment Plan (it was now just before dark) ?

Questions:

1. If satellite communications would allow a high risk night-time helicopter evacuation, would you take that option ?

2. What assessment elements might allow you to justify that decision ?

38

Assessment and Plan

A	A′	P
1900 Worsening ABD pain (w/ 36hr. Hx of ↑ discomfort)	volume shock	monitor vitals / cont. assessment
2000 Compensated volume shock (Hx: possible pregnancy)	decompensation	EVAC / monitor vitals

Notes:

What actually happened next...

The student complained of worsening focal pain and the rescuers monitored the pts. vitals with a pattern of increasing compensation during the hours the pt. remained in their care. The original plan was to attempt evacuation the following day but with the pts. dramatic deterioration, an evacuation was initiated at 0200hrs. and resulted in the pts. arrival at the hospital the following morning. The pt. went immediately into surgery and the diagnosis was an ectopic pregnancy with rupture which had resulted in a significant volume of internal bleeding.

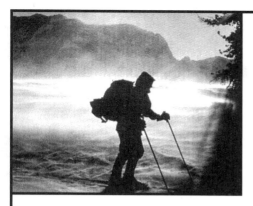

39 - FALL, SKIING
British Columbia

The story:

A group of young males, inspired by sunny weather, skied out of bounds to a remote area with a reputation for fine steep chute skiing. The conditions that day were as dangerous as ever likely to be encountered with the chutes sheathed in ice from days of a recent melt / freeze cycle. 2 of the individuals selected one of the steepest and tightest of the chutes as their descent route and both lost control immediately after skiing out onto the slope. Witnesses stated that the 2 picked up speed, lost their equipment, and started bouncing off trees in their path before disappearing into the bottom of the chute. The remaining skiers retraced their path out of bounds and reported the accident to ski patrollers on the nearest mtn. Although they responded immediately to the area below the chutes, it had been almost 45 minutes since the incident occurred when patrollers arrived on scene.

The first patrollers arrived at 1000hrs. to find one young male at the base of a tree.

On exam pt. #1: The pt. was unresponsive and after checking his carotid pulse for a full minute was determined to be in cardiac arrest.

As other patrollers arrived, the second pt. was discovered at the bottom of the chute, moaning with gurgling respirations.

On exam pt. #2: Pt. was pain responsive. His head had undergone significant trauma with deformity and swelling around the face and the posterior skull. Pt. had a significant amount of blood in the airway: this was immediately cleared and PPV initiated. The patient suffered from severe respiratory distress with crepitus noted in the L anterior and lateral chest wall. Breath sounds were absent on the L side. The abdomen was distended and tender. No gross deformities were noted in the extremities although the patient moaned loudly when his lower extremities were stabilized or moved. Circulation x 4 extremities.

Pt. #1: Despite CPR, remained in arrest, the pts. chest wall and skull were very unstable.

Pt. #2: The pts. pulse: 140 and weak, Resp.: 40 and extremely labored, B/P: 180/p, Skin: pale, cool, moist, Temp.: UTA, Pt. was P on AVPU

Put the appropriate information from the story above into the correct spaces in the SOAP note.

Develop an Assessment for 1000hrs. with Anticipated Problems and an appropriate Treatment Plan for both these patients.

The patrollers had access to ALS helicopter and ground ambulances. The evac. time from the scene after packaging was roughly 20 minutes to the base area and an additional 30 min. by air to the Trauma Center.

Question:

With 2 rescuers on scene, how would you manage these 2 pts.? With 3 rescuers ?

39

Assessment and Plan

A	**A'**	**P**
1000		
Pt.#1		
Cardiac arrest	cont. arrest	CPR / triage
Pt.#2		
Respiratory failure 2° blunt trauma to L lat. chest w/crepitus	respiratory arrest	PPV / EVAC. / ALS
Volume shock 2° internal bleed. w/ tender ABD	decompensation	Monitor / EVAC
↑ICP (P on AVPU) w/ severe head/ facial injury	cont. ↑ICP	Monitor esp. airway
Unable to clear spine 2* distracting injuries, ↓AVPU	swelling	Immobilize
Unstable ext. injuries	swelling / ischemia	Stabilize / monitor

Notes:

What actually happened next...

Pt. 2 was evacuated first to the base area, arriving in a toboggan behind a ski patroller travelling as fast as possible. By the time the toboggan arrived in the base area, a medical helicopter had landed and the pt. was taken directly to the LZ. The pts. chest was decompressed by the flight crew and the resp. distress improved dramatically. Additionally, an IV was established, various medications were administered, and the pt. was intubated. Pt. 1 arrived in the base area at about this time and resuscitation efforts were discontinued. Pt. 2 was flown immediately to a Level 1 Trauma Center and survived despite his injuries. In fact, this pt. recovered so well he returned (this time with a snowboard) the following season.

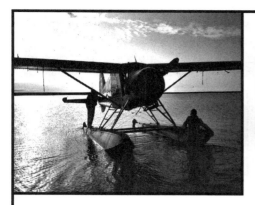

40 - PLANE CRASH
South Dakota

The story:

Note: the following is an exercise in triage. Assume you were one of the EMT's on scene and were responsible for making the decisions regarding patient treatment and evacuation. Develop a prioritized list of all patients on scene and then, following the parameters detailed below, make a decision as to whom to transport.

A twin engine aircraft with 7 passengers was chartered to return a group back home after a weekend meeting. The pilot tried to get through a mountain pass, but lost power and pancaked into a snow field at the 3000'(900m) level. The FAA picked up an ELT signal, and launched military and commercial helicopters. There were 2 EMT's equipped with a small jump kit and BLS supplies in a Bell 206 that initially found the wreckage. The weather was deteriorating and it was not clear if any other aircraft would be able to reach the crash site. The helicopter could carry a single stretcher patient or up to 3 patients sitting upright.

1 30 y/o fem., AOx4, sitting outside the wreckage, sustained a crush fx of the distal left tib/fib. with good CSM. **P:** 80, **R:** 14, **BP:** 130/80, **S:** warm.

2 Pilot, 40 y/o male, lying under left wing, moved from the cockpit by others. Awake and lethargic, c/o: difficulty breathing. Bruise on chest w/ crepitus in the ribs and decreased breath sounds on rt. Angulated open Fx of the R ankle. Lac. over L eye. **BP:** 140/80 **P:** 100, **R:** 30, shallow, **S:** pale, cool.

3 24 y/o female, Awake and groggy. This patient was standing upon arrival, c/o: pain in left chest and elbow, c/o feeling "cold". **P:** 50, **R:** 10, **BP:** 100/60, **S:** pale, cool..

4 51 y/o female, Awake and lethargic, shivering. Trapped in the wreckage for 90min., c/o: severe pain right hip. Exam shows deformity in pelvic region w/ unstable right femur. Open Fx left tib/fib. Deep lac. from bridge of nose to left cheek. **P:** 130, **R:** 36, **BP:** 110/70, **S:** pale, cool.

5 28 y/o male, Awake and anxious. Pt. is ambulatory on arrival. Exam shows 1"(2.5cm) laceration on chin and contusion on the rt. lower leg. **P:** 100, **R:** 20, **S:** normal.

6 34 y/o male. Supine in snow next to tail of the aircraft. No palp. pulse or respirations. Survivors dragged him from the wreckage, stating: "he was still alive a few minutes ago". Exam reveals an open crush fracture on the L side of the pts. forehead.

7 31 y/o male, Awake and anxious. Pt. is cold and shivering, c/o: left shoulder pain. Exam shows unstable left clavicle with obvious deformity. **P:** 120, **R:** 20 easy, **BP:** 150/80, **S:** pale, cool, moist,

Question:

Boy HOWDY! If it were doubtful that another helicopter could make it to the scene before the weather deteriorated and it was your decision, who would you transport and how in a small helicopter ?

Assessment and Plan

<u>A</u>	<u>A′</u>	<u>P</u>
triage order:		

Notes:

What actually happened next...

Once again, the situation was helped immeasurably by the availability of helicopter evacuation. All pts. were eventually transported by aircraft and the difficult decision of who got evacuated and who didn't never had to be made. These tough decisions have been made on much larger scale incidents than this plane crash in the past and will undoubtedly continue to be made in the future. It is helpful for student to know that, in most cases, the medical crew onboard the aircraft will make the decisions when it comes to triage and an example of that decision and the reasoning behind it follows:

Triage: the Greatest Good for the Greatest Number.

#1
pt.**2** (he is a critical pt. and could be positioned upright despite the MOI to help with his respiratory distress.)

#2
pt.**3** (her mental status and vitals in addition to the unspecified pain in her chest make her a priority candidate for evac.)

#3
pt.**7** (he has an unstable clavicle injury and it's proximity to vital structures in the chest as well as his vitals make this pt. a priority over pt.1)

These 3 could fly out with the first available aircraft. Pt. **4**, although critical, must fly in a supine position and therefore will have to wait for the second available aircraft.
Pts. **1** and **5** are stable at the time of assessment and although that could change over time, these folks will wait for evac. Pt. **6** will be evacuated last as his arrest was likely the result of trauma and his chances for recovery are nonexistent.
As a final note...Where is the last pt.? (you can imagine missing someone in a situation like this can't you?)

Thanks

This Workbook would not have been possible without the stories, insight, and support of Wilderness Medical Associates Instructors and office staff. This group of Physicians, EMT's, PA's, Nurses and Paramedics have proven to be some of the most professional, motivated, and helpful folks I have yet had the pleasure of working with.

For editorial input, many thanks to: Mary Beth Brandt, Lucca Criminale, Justin Grohs, Jeff Issac, and David Johnson.

For story submissions, thanks to: Rocco Altobelli, Jeff Baierlein, LeAnne Carson, Sherrie Collins, Lucca Criminale, Cynthia Flores, Bill Frederick, Justin Grohs, Steve Hahn, Jeff Issac, John Jacobs, Fay Johnson, Ron Johnson, David Johnson, Hilary Lauer, Maggie Handlan, Ray Martodam, Jim Morrissey, Mike Motti, Julie Nordyke, Chuck Rose, Nick Runions, Ellen Schafhauser, Georgia Villaflor, and Ben Woodard.

To all the many WMA instructors and office staff, many thanks,

Tom Clausing, Leavenworth, WA

Story Key

story #	primary focus	secondary focus	MOI / Sx	environment
1	blunt trauma	MOI spine	fall	on board ship
2	multi-systems trauma	musculoskeletal	fall	glissading
3	multi-systems trauma	spine injury	hits trees	skiing
4	blunt chest trauma	MOI spine	fall	from horse
5	asthma	Hx	distress	portaging
6	facial burns	evacuation	burns	cooking
7	respiratory arrest	near drowning	failed roll	kayaking
8	concussion	spine protocol	fall	mt. biking
9	concussion	evacuation	fall	hunting
10	↑ ICP	evacuation	fall	scrambling
11	trauma arrest	↑ ICP	fall	traverse
12	spine protocol	ASR	fall	descending
13	spine injury / deficit	evacuation	fall	rock climbing
14	cervical spine injury	evacuation	avalanche	climbing
15	stable vs. unstable	ASR	slip	stream crossing
16	unstable leg	evacuation	wash over falls	kayaking
17	unstable pelvis	multi-systems trauma	fall	off cornice
18	shoulder protocol	Hx	wet exit	kayaking
19	toxin ingestion	volume shock	NVD	hiking
20	anaphylaxis protocol	Hx	bee sting	paddling
21	snake bite	evacuation	snake bite	hiking
22	scorpion sting	local / systemic toxin	sting	rafting
23	burn management	infection / evacuation	cooking burn	canyoneering
24	wound protocol	wilderness vs. hospital	bite	snorkeling
25	wound protocol	wilderness vs. hospital	bear attack	hiking
26	severe hypothermia	near drowning	broach	canoeing
27	severe hypothermia	evacuation	winter	backpacking
28	heat exhaustion	hyponatremia	exhaustion	hiking
29	heat stroke	STOPEATS	seizure	hiking
30	hyponatremia	STOPEATS	cramps	hiking
31	hypoglycemia	STOPEATS	weakness	biking
32	seizure	STOPEATS / evacuation	seizure	backpacking
33	HACE	STOPEATS / evacuation	ataxia	climbing
34	lightning: cardiac / resp.	burns	lightning	backpacking
35	frostbite	evacuation	exposure	climbing
36	HAPE	evacuation	distress	altitude
37	GI infection	volume shock	GI distress	trekking
38	ABD pain	volume shock	ABD pain	rafting
39	MCI / triage	multi-systems trauma	fall	skiing
40	MCI / triage	evacuation	plane crash	mountains

NOTES

NOTES

NOTES

NOTES